Diagnosis and Management of Type II Diabetes

First Edition

Steven V. Edelman, MD
Associate Professor of Medicine
Division of Endocrinology and Metabolism
University of California, San Diego

Robert R. Henry, MD
Professor of Medicine
Division of Endocrinology and Metabolism
University of California, San Diego

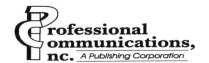

Professional
Communications,
Inc. *A Publishing Corporation*

Copyright 1997
Steven V. Edelman, MD
and Robert R. Henry, MD

Published by:
Professional Communications, Inc.

All rights reserved. No part of this publication may be reproduced or transmitted in any form or by any means, electronic or mechanical, including photocopy, recording or any other information storage and retrieval system, without the prior agreement and written permission of the publisher. Requests for permission or further information should be addressed to Professional Communications, Inc.; P.O. Box 10; Caddo, OK 74729-0010 or faxed to 405/367-9989.

For orders only, please call:
1-800-337-9838

ISBN: 1-884735-13-4

Printed in the United States of America

This text is printed on recycled paper.

DEDICATION

To our wives, Ingrid and Denine,
and our children, Talia, Carina,
Ryan, Danny and Dustin,
for their tolerance and patience during
the writing of this book.

ACKNOWLEDGMENT

The basis for this book has come from the hard work of diabetes specialists dedicated to helping people with diabetes live healthier and happier lives. Individuals such as Mayer Davidson, Richard Berkson, Alain Baron, Irl Hirsh, Jim Dudl, Joan Fitzgerald, and Ingrid Kruse are just a fraction of the gentle and sometimes silent giants devoted to the field of diabetes.

We would like also to express our appreciation to Karen Lloyd for her assistance in medical writing, Phyllis Freeny for her excellent editorial assistance, and Nikki D. Stewart for her exceptional graphics design work. Our secretaries, Sherri Williams and Betsy Hansen, were also invaluable sources of help. Lastly, we would like to thank Malcolm Beasley for his patience and unyielding support in writing this book.

TABLE OF CONTENTS

TABLES

FIGURES

1   Diabetes Statistics

Diabetes is a serious disease that can have a significant impact on the health, quality of life, and life expectancy of individuals, as well as on the health-care system. Approximately 16 million men, women, and children in the United States have diabetes (10% have type I and 90% have type II diabetes), representing about 6% of the total population.[1] Eight million of these individuals have been diagnosed with diabetes; the other 8 million are undiagnosed and may be unaware that they have this disorder.[1,2] Many of these individuals are asymptomatic for years and often have developed diabetic complications before a diagnosis is made.

Prevalence and Incidence of Type II Diabetes

■ Prevalence of Type II Diabetes

The prevalence of diabetes increases with age, as shown in Figure 1.1. For the years 1991-1993, the mean percentage of people with diagnosed diabetes increased substantially from 0.8% in the under 45-year-old age group to 5.8% in the 45- to 64-year-old age group.[1] Another striking increase occurred in the 45- to 64-year-old age group compared with the 65- to 74-year-old age group (5.8% to 10.7%, respectively).[1]

Gender differences in the prevalence of diagnosed diabetes also can be observed in Figure 1.1. Women have a slightly higher prevalence than men (55% vs 45%, respectively).[1] These differences are more readily observed at a national level and less apparent in smaller databases such as the community, in part because of

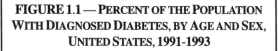

FIGURE 1.1 — PERCENT OF THE POPULATION WITH DIAGNOSED DIABETES, BY AGE AND SEX, UNITED STATES, 1991-1993

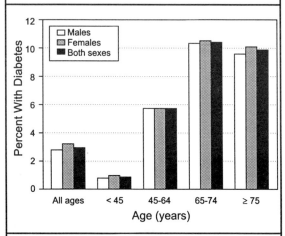

Data are the average for the 3 years 1991-1993.

Source: Kenny SJ, Aubert RE, Geiss LS. Prevalence and incidence of non–insulin-dependent diabetes. In: Harris MI, Cowie CC, Stern MP, et al, eds. *Diabetes in America*, 2nd ed. Bethesda, Md: National Institutes of Health, National Institutes of Diabetes and Digestive and Kidney Diseases; 1995:50-53. NIH Publ. No. 95-1468.

variations in risk factors, such as obesity or genetic composition.

Racial and ethnic variations in the prevalence of diagnosed and undiagnosed diabetes in the United States are shown in Table 1.1. A disproportionate prevalence of diabetes exists among African Americans, Hispanic Americans, and American Indians.

The Pima Indians of Arizona have the highest rate of diabetes in the world. Approximately 50% of the population between ages 30 and 64 years of age have

TABLE 1.1 — PERCENTAGE OF ADULTS WITH DIABETES BY RACE AND ETHNICITY

Ethnic/Racial Group	% With Diabetes
African Americans	9.6
Mexican Americans	9.6
Cuban Americans	9.1
Puerto Rican Americans	10.9
Caucasian Americans	6.2
American Indians	5.0-50.0

Source: Centers for Disease Control. National Diabetes Fact Sheet (National estimates released November, 1995). Atlanta, Ga: CDC Diabetes Home Page (http://www.cdc.gov/nccdphp/ddt/facts.htm).

type II diabetes. A high prevalence of type II diabetes also exists among other Native American groups.[1]

The overall prevalence of diabetes (type I and type II) has increased steadily over the last 35 years (Figure 1.2).

The 3% rate reported for the years 1991-1993 is more than three times the rate in 1960 (0.9%) and eight times the rate in 1935 (0.4%).[1] Several possible reasons for the substantial increases over time include:

- Increasing age of the US population (diabetes prevalence increases with age)
- Reduction in mortality rates of people with diabetes because of improved screening, detection, and health care
- Increase in risk factors such as:
  - Degree of obesity
  - Physical inactivity.

In the United States, the prevalence of undiagnosed type II diabetes is approximately equal to the

FIGURE 1.2 — TIME TRENDS IN THE NUMBER AND
PERCENT OF THE POPULATION WITH DIAGNOSED
DIABETES (IDDM AND NIDDM), UNITED STATES,
1958-1993

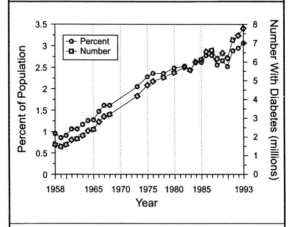

Source: Kenny SJ, Aubert RE, Geiss LS. Prevalence and
incidence of non–insulin-dependent diabetes. In: Harris MI,
Cowie CC, Stern MP, et al, eds. *Diabetes in America*, 2nd ed.
Bethesda, Md: National Institutes of Health, National
Institutes of Diabetes and Digestive and Kidney Diseases;
1995:50-53. NIH Publ. No. 95-1468.

rate of diagnosed type II diabetes.[1-2] Consequently,
the actual prevalence of diabetes is twice the rate of
diagnosed diabetes. In addition, 10% to 15% of people
age 50 years and older are estimated to have undiagnosed type II diabetes. When age adjustments are
taken into consideration, the rate of undiagnosed diabetes is 1.5 times higher in African Americans and 1.7
times higher in Mexican Americans than in Caucasians.

Undiagnosed type II diabetes threatens the health
of many people, particularly because complications are
likely to develop the longer that diabetes goes unrecognized and untreated. For example, retinopathy has

been observed in 20% of individuals with undiagnosed type II diabetes at the time of their initial diagnosis.[1] Higher rates of macrovascular complications (stroke, angina, myocardial infarction) also are common at the time of diagnosis in people with previously undiagnosed type II diabetes.

■ Incidence of Type II Diabetes

Data for 1990 to 1992 suggest that approximately 625,000 people are diagnosed with diabetes each year.[1-2] Nearly half of the new cases are found in people age 55 years and older, and more women are diagnosed than men (58% vs 42%, respectively).[1] The average annual incidence rate in the United States in 1990 to 1992 was 2.4 per 1000 people.

Although incidence rates increased during the 1960s, they were more stable from 1968 through 1992. The 1990 to 1992 incidence rate of 2.4 per 1000 was 1.4 times the rate in 1964 (1.8 per 1000) and 6.4 times the rate in 1935 to 1936 (0.4 per 1000).[1]

Ethnic/racial variations in incidence of diabetes are similar to the prevalence rates in these populations. African Americans, Hispanics, and Native Americans have a higher incidence rate than Caucasians.

Mortality in Type II Diabetes

A significant number of deaths in the United States each year can be attributed to diabetes. In 1993, approximately 400,000 deaths from all causes were reported in people with diabetes.[2] This figure represents 18% of all deaths in the United States in people age 25 years and older.

According to the National Center for Health Statistics,[2] diabetes was the seventh leading cause of death listed on US death certificates in 1993, and the sixth leading cause of death by disease type. Based on death leading cause of death by disease type. Based on death certificate data,[1] diabetes is the:

- Fourth leading cause of death in African American women
- Third leading cause of death in:
  - Hispanic women ages 45 to 74 years
  - Native American women ages 65 to 74 years.

Higher mortality rates in these racial/ethnic groups are partially related to the higher prevalance of diabetes in these populations.

Having type II diabetes reduces the life expectancy of middle-aged people by approximately 5 to 10 years, although this number decreases as a person ages.[1] Women tend to lose more years of life expectancy than men, particularly when they are diagnosed at a young age. Having complications of type II diabetes also reduces life expectancy.

The leading causes of death according to the death certificates of people with diabetes are shown in Figure 1.3. People with diabetes are 2 to 4 times more likely to die from heart disease than people without diabetes.[1,2] This risk exists regardless of age and the presence of other risk factors. Excess risk of cardiovascular mortality exists in younger people as well as:

- Older people with diabetes
- Those with younger onset and longer duration
- Those using insulin
- Women.

The presence of complications in people with type II diabetes also increases their risk of death. Other factors that influence the risk of early death in type II diabetes, which are similar for people with type I diabetes, are:

- Duration of diabetes
- Lack of blood glucose control
- Cardiovascular risk factors such as:

14

FIGURE 1.3 — APPROXIMATE DISTRIBUTION OF CAUSES OF DEATH IN PEOPLE WITH DIABETES, BASED ON US STUDIES

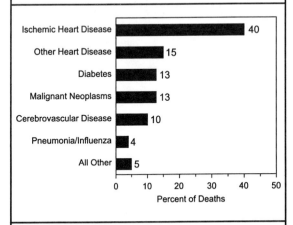

Source: Geiss LS, Herman WH, Smith PJ. Mortality in non–insulin-dependent diabetes. In: Harris MI, Cowie CC, Stern MP, et al, eds. *Diabetes in America*. Bethesda, Md: National Institutes of Health, National Institutes of Diabetes and Digestive and Kidney Diseases; 1995:236-237.

– Smoking
– Hypertension
– Abnormal lipid levels
– Physical inactivity
– Central obesity.

REFERENCES

1. American Diabetes Association. *Diabetes 1996 Vital Statistics*. Alexandria, Va: American Diabetes Association; 1996.

2. National Institutes of Diabetes and Digestive and Kidney Diseases. *Diabetes Statistics*. Bethesda, Md: NIDDK, 1995; NIH publication no. 96-3926 (http://www.niddk.nih.gov/DiabetesStatistics/DiabetesStatistics.html).

Additional Reading

National Diabetes Data Group. *Diabetes in America*, 2nd ed. Bethesda, Md: National Institutes of Health; 1995. NIH Publication No. 95-1468.

2 Pathophysiology

Type II diabetes is known to have a strong genetic component with contributing environmental determinants.[1] The genetic influence is strongly evidenced by data from twin and family studies.[2-6] Identification of type II diabetes susceptibility genes has been elusive, and investigations of a number of candidate genes has been largely negative, yielding a very small population of patients (less than 5%) with genetic variation in any of the candidate genes studied to date.

It is likely that no single genetic defect will emerge to explain type II diabetes; thus, the disease is heterogeneous and possibly multigenetic, and likely has a complex etiology. Even though the disease is genetically heterogeneous, there appears to be a fairly consistent phenotype once the disease is fully manifested. Most patients with type II diabetes and fasting hyperglycemia are characterized by:

- Insulin resistance
- Impaired insulin secretion
- Increased hepatic glucose production.[7-11]

Although these three metabolic abnormalities have been well studied and characterized, the etiologic sequence has only recently come into focus.

It is clear that the increased hepatic glucose production of type II diabetes is secondary and can be fully reversed with a variety of forms of antidiabetic therapy.[12-14] In addition, increased hepatic glucose production rates do not exist in the state of impaired glucose tolerance (IGT).[12] This leaves insulin resistance, impaired insulin secretion, or both, as initiating abnormalities.

Recent accumulated evidence strongly supports the idea that insulin resistance, not impaired insulin secretion, precedes the onset of hyperglycemia and the type II diabetes phenotype.[15-16] In fact, studies have also shown that insulin secretion, including first-phase insulin responses to intravenous glucose, are either normal or increased in the prediabetic or IGT state.[7,10-11] Thus, substantial evidence from the literature indicates that those individuals who evolve to type II diabetes from IGT begin with insulin resistance.

In addition to the idea that insulin resistance is likely to be a primary inherited feature in most patients with type II diabetes, acquired features may also be contributory, such as:

- Obesity
- Sedentary lifestyle
- Aging.

If beta cell function is normal, this will lead to hyperinsulinemia, which maintains relatively normal glucose tolerance. Therefore, in the compensated insulin-resistant, hyperinsulinemic state, one has either normal glucose tolerance or impaired glucose tolerance, but not diabetes. A subpopulation of individuals with compensated insulin resistance eventually go on to develop type II diabetes. The magnitude of this subpopulation depends on the means of detecting glucose intolerance, particular ethnic groups studied, and several other acquired and metabolic abnormalities that may be present. In addition, during the transition from the compensated state to frank type II diabetes, at least three pathophysiologic changes can be observed:

- First, basal hepatic glucose production rates increase, which is a characteristic feature of essentially all type II diabetes patients with fasting hyperglycemia.[7-11]
- Second, the insulin resistance usually becomes more severe, which may be due to the degree of

genetic load and/or acquired conditions such as obesity, sedentary lifestyle, and aging.[15,17] Antidiabetic treatment can completely normalize the elevated hepatic glucose production rates and partially ameliorate the insulin resistance so that the degree of insulin resistance returns approximately to the level present in the IGT state. Thus, increased hepatic output and the worsening of insulin resistance are likely to be secondary phenomena.

- The third and most marked change is a decrease in beta cell function and decline in insulin secretory ability. Whether this decline in insulin secretion is because of preprogrammed genetic abnormalities in beta cell function or acquired defects such as glucose toxicity or beta cell exhaustion, or both, remains to be elucidated. Nevertheless, a marked decrease in beta cell function accompanies this transition and is thought to be a major contributor to the transition from IGT to type II diabetes.

In summary, the proposed etiologic sequence is that insulin resistance (either genetic or acquired) is manifested initially, leading to increased insulin secretion to maintain the compensated IGT state. In time, the compensation fails and beta cell function declines, leading to hyperglycemia. In addition, the conversion of IGT to type II diabetes can also be influenced by:

- Ethnicity
- Degree of obesity
- Distribution of body fat
- Sedentary lifestyle
- Aging
- Other concomitant medical conditions.

The heterogeneous nature of type II diabetes and its natural history result in the varied response to the different antidiabetic agents over time.

REFERENCES

1. Hamman RF. Genetic and environmental determinations of non–insulin-dependent diabetes mellitus (NIDDM). *Diabetes Metab Rev*. 1992;8:287-338.

2. O'Rahilly S, Wainscoat JS, Turner RC. Type 2 (non–insulin-dependent) diabetes mellitus. New genetics for old nightmares. *Diabetologia*. 1988;31:407-414.

3. Rich SS. Mapping genes in diabetes: genetic epidemiological perspective. *Diabetes*. 1990;39:1315-1319.

4. Permutt MA. Genetics of NIDDM. *Diabetes Care*. 1990;13: 1150-1153.

5. Granner DK, O'Brien RM. Molecular physiology and genetics of NIDDM. Importance of metabolic staging. *Diabetes Care*. 1992;15:369-395.

6. Kobberling J, Tillil H. Genetic and nutritional factors in the etiology and pathogenesis of diabetes mellitus. *World Rev Nutr Diet*. 1990;63:102-115.

7. Olefsky JM. Etiology and pathogenesis of non–insulin-dependent diabetes (type II). In: *DeGroot: Endocrinology*, 2nd ed. New York: Grune and Stratton, Inc; 1989:1369-1388.

8. DeFronzo RA. Lilly lecture 1987. The triumvirate: beta-cell, muscle, liver. A collusion responsible for NIDDM. *Diabetes*. 1988;37:667-687.

9. Reaven GM. Banting lecture. Role of insulin resistance in human disease. *Diabetes*. 1988;37:1595-1607.

10. Seely BL, Olefsky JM. Potential cellular and genetic mechanisms for insulin resistance in common disorders of obesity and diabetes. In: Moller D, ed. *Insulin Resistance and Its Clinical Disorders*. London: John Wiley & Sons, Ltd; 1993: 187-252.

11. Olefsky JM. Insulin resistance and the pathogenesis of non–insulin-dependent diabetes mellitus: cellular and molecular mechanisms. In: Efendic S, Ostenson CG, Vranic M, eds. *New Concepts in the Pathogenesis of NIDDM*. New York: Plenum Publishing Corporation; 1995.

12. Henry RR, Gumbiner B, Ditzler ST, Wallace P, Lyon R, Glauber HS. Intensive conventional insulin therapy for type II diabetes: metabolic effects during a 6-month outpatient trial. *Diabetes Care*. 1993;16:21-31.

13. Henry RR, Wallace P, Olefsky JM. Effects of weight loss on mechanisms of hyperglycemia in obese non–insulin-dependent diabetes mellitus. *Diabetes*. 1986;35:990-998.

14. Garvey WT, Olefsky JM, Griffin J, Hammon R, Kolterman OG. The effects of insulin treatment on insulin secretion and action in type II diabetes mellitus. *Diabetes*. 1985;34:222-234.

15. Eriksson J, Franssila-Kallunki A, Ekstrand A, et al. Early metabolic defects in persons at increased risk for non–insulin-dependent diabetes mellitus. *N Engl J Med*. 1989;321:337-343.

16. Warram JH, Martin BC, Krolewski AS, Soeldner JS, Kahn CR. Slow glucose removal rate and hyperinsulinemia precede the development of type II diabetes in the offspring of diabetic parents. *Ann Intern Med*. 1990;113:909-915.

17. DeFronzo RA, Ferrannini E. Insulin resistance. A multi-faceted syndrome responsible for NIDDM, obesity, hypertension, dyslipidemia and atherosclerotic cardiovascular disease. *Diabetes Care*. 1991;14:173-194.

3   Classification

Diabetes mellitus and other categories of glucose intolerance can be divided into three main clinical categories:

- Diabetes mellitus (with four clinical subclasses)
- Impaired glucose tolerance (IGT)
- Gestational diabetes mellitus (GDM).

The common denominator of a group of disorders that constitute the syndrome of diabetes mellitus is fasting hyperglycemia or plasma glucose levels above the limits established by the National Diabetes Data Group (NDDG).[1] The four subclasses of diabetes mellitus are:

- Type I diabetes mellitus (insulin-dependent)
- Type II diabetes mellitus (non–insulin-dependent)
- Secondary/other types of diabetes associated with certain conditions
- Malnutrition-related diabetes mellitus.

Each of these subclasses has distinctive characteristics (Table 3.1).

Type I Diabetes Mellitus

Type 1 diabetes is defined by the presence of ketosis caused by an almost complete lack of insulin or severe insulinopenia. Immunologic destruction of the beta cells is the etiologic basis of type I diabetes. An autoimmune cause is suggested by evidence of circulating antibodies to islet cells, to endogenous insulin, and/or to other antigen components of islet cells at the time of diagnosis. Patients commonly are lean and

TABLE 3.1 — DISTINGUISHING CHARACTERISTICS OF DIABETES MELLITUS AND OTHER DISORDERS OF GLUCOSE INTOLERANCE

Category	Distinguishing Characteristics
Diabetes Mellitus	
Type I diabetes (insulin-dependent)	Any age, usually not obese, often abrupt onset, signs/symptoms usually before age 20, positive urine ketone test with hyperglycemia, insulin therapy necessary to sustain life and prevent ketoacidosis
Type II diabetes (non-insulin-dependent)	Usually over age 30 at diagnosis, obese, few classic symptoms, not prone to ketoacidosis unless under severe physical stress (eg, infection), exogenous insulin usually not needed to control hyperglycemia for many years
Secondary/Other Types of Diabetes Mellitus	
Secondary to pancreatic disease	Pancreatectomy, hemochromatosis, cystic fibrosis, chronic pancreatitis

Secondary to endocrinopathies	Cushing's syndrome, acromegaly, pheochromocytoma, primary aldosteronism, glucagonoma
Secondary to drugs and chemical agents	Certain antihypertensive drugs (thiazides, diuretics, or β-blockers), glucocorticoids, estrogen-containing preparations, nicotinic acid, phenytoin, catecholamines
Associated with insulin receptor abnormalities	Acanthosis nigricans
Associated with genetic syndromes	Lipodystrophic syndromes, muscular dystrophies, Huntington's chorea
Associated with miscellaneous conditions	Polycystic ovary disease
Malnutrition-related diabetes mellitus	Young age (10 to 40), usually symptomatic, not prone to ketoacidosis, most require insulin therapy
Impaired glucose tolerance (IGT)	Plasma glucose levels are higher than normal but not diagnostic of diabetes mellitus
Gestational diabetes mellitus (GDM)	Onset or discovery of glucose intolerance during pregnancy

Source: Adapted from American Diabetes Association. *Medical Management of Non-insulin-dependent (Type II) Diabetes*; 3rd ed. Alexandria, Va: American Diabetes Association; 1994.

have experienced considerable weight loss; almost all are diagnosed before age 20 years, although type I diabetes can develop at any age. Approximately 10% of all individuals who have been diagnosed with diabetes have type I diabetes.[2] Daily insulin injections are required throughout the patient's life to prevent ketoacidosis and death.

Type II Diabetes Mellitus

Type II diabetes is the most common type of diabetes, accounting for 85% to 90% of all diagnosed cases in the United States, and is more prevalent among various non-Caucasian ethnic/racial populations, such as American Indians, African Americans, Pacific Islanders, and Hispanics.[3] A strong genetic basis exists for type II diabetes (approximately 90% of patients with type II diabetes have a positive family history of this disorder). In addition, identical twin studies have revealed a 60% to 90% concordance for diabetes.[3] An absence of ketosis is one of the primary features that distinguishes type II diabetes from type I diabetes, although it is possible to have ketonemia with type II diabetes.

Patients with type II diabetes can vary considerably in their ability to secrete insulin. Insulin secretion, however, is inadequate to overcome the insulin resistance associated with this type of diabetes. Defects of insulin action (insulin resistance) are typical of type II diabetes.

Obesity is strongly associated with type II diabetes. Approximately 90% of people with type II diabetes are obese (20% over ideal body weight)[3] and the chances of developing type II diabetes double for every 20% increase in body weight in susceptible individuals.[2] However, type II diabetes also can develop in nonobese individuals; this is more commonly observed in older patients. The incidence of type II dia-

26

betes increases with age and obesity in part because people tend to gain weight and especially develop central abdominal obesity as they age.

Type II diabetes usually is diagnosed after the age of 40, although it may be diagnosed more frequently at a younger age (eg, 30 years old) in certain ethnic groups prone to developing diabetes. Patients are usually asymptomatic and only occasionally display the classic symptoms of diabetes mellitus (polydipsia, polyuria, polyphagia, weight loss). Because type II diabetes can go unrecognized for many years, early stages of microvascular disease and frank macrovascular complications may be present by the time a diagnosis is made.

Secondary/Other Types of Diabetes Mellitus

This smallest category of diabetes mellitus includes diabetes related to certain other diseases, conditions, or drugs. Hyperglycemia is present at a level that is diagnostic of diabetes. Patients are placed in this category if their diabetes has a known or probable cause or is part of a specific condition or syndrome (Table 3.1). Treatment of the underlying disorder may ameliorate the diabetes; more frequently, however, it is necessary to treat the diabetes with diet, exercise, and medications.

Malnutrition-related Diabetes Mellitus

This type of diabetes is seen for the most part in developing countries and tends to affect young individuals between 10 and 40 years old. The classic symptoms of hyperglycemia are present without ketoacidosis, and insulin usually is required to control hyperglycemia. The role of malnutrition as a causal factor is unknown.

Impaired Glucose Tolerance

Individuals who have plasma glucose levels that are higher than normal but lower than established diagnostic values for diabetes mellitus are classified as having IGT (diagnostic criteria in Table 3.2). This condition is common (approximately 11% of the US population) and considered a precursor of type II diabetes. Although individuals with IGT are more likely to eventually develop diabetes mellitus, only approximately 25% do develop type II diabetes and a similar percentage subsequently have normal glucose levels. The rate of progression is approximately 5% to 10% per year and can be influenced by:

TABLE 3.2 — DIAGNOSTIC CRITERIA FOR IMPAIRED GLUCOSE TOLERANCE (IGT) USING THE ORAL GLUCOSE TOLERANCE TEST (OGTT)*

World Health Organization criteria		
IGT	**Old**	**New**
Fasting	< 140	< 126
and 2-h	140-199	140-199
Diabetes		
Fasting	> 140	> 126
and 2-h	$\geq$ 200	$\geq$ 200
National Diabetes Data Group criteria		
IGT		
Fasting	< 140	
and 2-h	140-199	
and one intermediate value	$\geq$ 200	
(at 0.5-, 1.0-, or 1.5-h)		

* 75-g glucose load.

Source: Edelman SV. Impaired glucose tolerance: a precursor of NIDDM or a disease entity in itself? *Diabetes News.* 1995;16:1-8.

- Ethnic origin
- Degree of obesity
- Distribution of body fat
- Sedentary lifestyle
- Aging
- Concomitant medical conditions.

Individuals with IGT are more susceptible to macro-vascular disease (coronary artery, peripheral vascular, cerebrovascular), which often is present at the time of diagnosis. Pharmacologic therapies and nonpharmacologic interventions such as weight reduction, improved diet, and increased physical activity may prevent the progression of IGT to type II diabetes by reducing insulin resistance.

Gestational Diabetes Mellitus

Glucose intolerance that is first detected during pregnancy is classified as GDM. Excluded from this group are women who had diabetes before conception. GDM occurs in about 2% to 4% of pregnant women, usually during the second or third trimester, and is more common in women who are older, obese, or have a family history of diabetes. This condition is important to identify because of the increased risk of fetal morbidity and mortality with GDM. Pregnant women should be screened with a 50-g, 1-hour glucose tolerance test during the 24th to 28th weeks of pregnancy. Approximately 81% to 94% of women with GDM return to normal glucose tolerance after delivery.[2] However, women who have had GDM are at increased risk of developing type II diabetes, with approximately 30% to 40% developing type II diabetes or IGT within 10 to 20 years.[2]

Problems With Classification

Sometimes it is difficult to distinguish between type I and type II diabetes. For example, younger type II patients who are thin and taking insulin may resemble type I patients. In addition, some patients display the characteristics of type II diabetes and are not susceptible to ketoacidosis, yet they are taking insulin. These patients should not be classified as type I based solely on their insulin regimen, because they are taking insulin for glycemic control rather than as a life-sustaining therapy to prevent ketoacidosis and death.

Type II diabetes sometimes is found in children or adolescents, who usually are above their ideal body weight, as are most type II adults. One type of diabetes found in the pediatric population is called maturity-onset diabetes of the young (MODY) and is an example of an autosomal dominant form of inheritance of diabetes. Age alone should not be considered the diagnostic variable in these patients; they should be classified as having type II and not type I diabetes.

Another classification problem that can occur involves older patients who develop ketosis-prone, type I diabetes. The onset of this form of diabetes is slower in older adults and may resemble type II diabetes for a considerable amount of time. These individuals tend to be at or slightly below their ideal weight and respond poorly to oral antidiabetic agents. Ketones in their urine indicate a true lack of insulin. The insulin requirements thus become obvious and insulin therapy must be started to avoid severe ketoacidosis, coma, and death. These patients are more insulin sensitive than their obese counterparts with type II diabetes and require less insulin to control their diabetes.

REFERENCES

1. National Diabetes Data Group. Classification and diagnosis of diabetes mellitus and other categories of glucose intolerance. *Diabetes*. 1979;28:1039-1057.

2. Davidson MB. *Diabetes Mellitus: Diagnosis and Treatment*. 3rd ed. New York: Churchill Livingstone; 1991.

3. American Diabetes Association. *Diabetes 1996 Vital Statistics*. Alexandria, Va: American Diabetes Association; 1996.

3

4 Diagnosis

A diagnosis of diabetes can be suspected in the presence of the following signs and symptoms of hyperglycemia:
- Polydipsia (increased thirst)
- Polyuria (increased urinary frequency with increased volume)
- Fatigue
- Polyphagia (increased appetite)
- Weight loss
- Abnormal healing
- Blurred vision
- Increased occurrence of infections, particularly those caused by yeast.

Only a minority of adults who are diagnosed with diabetes are symptomatic initially. Consequently, the onset of type II diabetes may occur years before a diagnosis is made. Individuals who are asymptomatic tend to be diagnosed during a routine physical examination, treatment for another condition, or through specific diabetes screening. The risk of diabetes is increased in asymptomatic individuals if any of the following risk factors are present:
- A strong family history of diabetes (parents or sibling)
- Obesity (20% above ideal body weight), particularly central adiposity
- Certain races (American Indian, Hispanic, African, or Pacific Islander ancestry)
- Women with previous gestational diabetes or history of babies of 9 pounds or more at birth

- Previously identified impaired glucose tolerance (IGT)
- Hypertension or significant hypertriglyceridemia (> 250 mg/dL)
- 40 years of age with any of the preceding factors

Measuring plasma glucose concentrations is currently the only way to confirm a diagnosis of diabetes. Normal plasma glucose values[1] are presented in Table 4.1 and the criteria for diagnosing diabetes in nonpregnant adults[2] are shown in Table 4.2.

Three approaches to glucose testing can be used to diagnose diabetes:
- Fasting plasma glucose measurements
- Random plasma glucose measurements
- Oral glucose tolerance testing (OGTT).

The fasting plasma glucose test is the diagnostic test of choice and is used to diagnose approximately 90% of all individuals with type II diabetes.[2] Plasma glucose testing may be performed in individuals who have had food or beverages shortly before the test. This type of testing is referred to as random plasma glucose testing. An OGTT measuring only the fasting and 2-hour blood glucose can give excellent diagnostic data and is fairly easy to perform. Because the glycosylated hemoglobin test has not been standardized, it is not currently used for diagnosing diabetes.

Regardless of the type of test used, all abnormal laboratory values should be documented at least twice to avoid a misdiagnosis caused by laboratory errors, unless all values are extremely high or classic symptoms are present. An OGTT generally is not necessary for diagnosing diabetes. However, OGTT can be useful for evaluating high-risk individuals so that preventive measures can be started (diet modification, exercise, weight loss) at an early stage. The National

TABLE 4.1 — NORMAL PLASMA GLUCOSE VALUES FOR NONPREGNANT ADULTS

Fasting	Time zero	< 115 mg/dL (6.4 mM)
After 75-g oral glucose load	30 min	< 200 mg/dL (11.1 mM)
	60 min	< 200 mg/dL (11.1 mM)
	90 min	< 200 mg/dL (11.1 mM)
	120 min	< 140 mg/dL (7.8 mM)

Source: American Diabetes Association. *Diabetes 1996 Vital Statistics.* Alexandria, Va: American Diabetes Association; 1996.

TABLE 4.2 — NEW CRITERIA FOR DIAGNOSING DIABETES IN NONPREGNANT ADULTS

One or more of the following must be present:

• Fasting plasma glucose value of ≥ 126 mg/dL or greater on at least two separate occasions

• Random plasma glucose level of ≥ 200 mg/dL or greater with signs and symptoms of diabetes

• Fasting plasma glucose level < 126 mg/dL but a 2-hour glucose concentration of ≥ 200 mg/dL during a 75-gram oral glucose tolerance test

Diabetes Data Group (NDDG) and the World Health Organization (WHO) have prepared criteria for diagnosing diabetes mellitus and IGT based on OGTT (see Table 3.2).

Concerning pregnancy and OGTT, the recommended screening during the 24th to 28th weeks of gestation involves giving a 50-g glucose load without regard to the time of the last meal or the time of day. A 1-hour plasma glucose concentration of 140 mg/dL is considered a positive reading that calls for a formal OGTT with a 100-g glucose load and sampling before the glucose challenge and at 1, 2, and 3 hours after glucose challenge.[2-3]

A complete medical evaluation is indicated following a positive diagnostic blood test for diabetes. Patients should not be diagnosed on the basis of age alone. The purpose of this evaluation is to:

- Appropriately classify the patient
- Detect any underlying diseases that may require further evaluation
- Determine whether any of the complications of diabetes are present.

Table 4.3 shows a Diabetes Warranty Program developed as a reference for patients, outlining evaluations at every visit and annually. Getting patients involved in their own care is an important tool to improve compliance and motivation.

REFERENCES

1. American Diabetes Association. *Medical Management of Non–insulin-dependent (Type II) Diabetes*, 3rd ed. Alexandria, Va: American Diabetes Association; 1994.

2. Davidson MB. *Diabetes Mellitus: Diagnosis and Treatment*, 3rd ed. New York: Churchill Livingstone; 1991.

3. American Diabetes Association. *Diabetes 1996 Vital Statistics*. Alexandria, Va: American Diabetes Association; 1996.

4

TABLE 4.3 — DIABETES WARRANTY PROGRAM

What should be done at every visit?

	Date	Result	Date	Result	Date	Result	Date	Result
Weight								
Blood Pressure								
Foot Exam								
Glycohemoglobin Test								

What tests/exams should be done every year?

	Date	Result	Date	Result	Date	Result
Lipoprotein Profile (fasting) (HDL, LDL, TRG, Total CH)						
Urine Protein/Microalbumin						

Serum Creatinine /Creatinine Clearance					
Eye Exam					
Dental Exam					
Other Tests/Exams (depending on individual needs)					
Cardiologist (for heart disease)					
Podiatrist (for foot problems)					
Thyroid Function Tests					

Abbreviations: HDL, high-density lipoprotein; LDL, low-density lipoprotein; TRG, triglyceride; CH, cholesterol.

Source: Edelman SV. Diabetes Warranty Program. VA Endocrinology Clinic, VA Hospital, UCSD, La Jolla, California.

4

5 Nutrition

Nutrition Therapy

The most fundamental component of the diabetes treatment plan for all patients with type II diabetes is medical nutrition therapy. Specific goals of nutrition therapy in type II diabetes are to:[1]

- Achieve and maintain as near-normal blood glucose levels as possible by balancing food intake with physical activity, supplemented by oral hypoglycemic agents or insulin (endogenous or exogenous) as needed
- Normalize blood pressure
- Normalize serum lipid levels
- Help patients attain and maintain a reasonable body weight (defined as the weight an individual and health-care provider acknowledge as possible to achieve and maintain on a short- and long-term basis)
- Promote overall health through optimal nutrition and lifestyle behaviors.

Because no single dietary approach is appropriate for all patients, given the heterogeneous nature of type II diabetes, meal plans and diet modifications should be individualized to meet a patient's unique needs and lifestyle. Accordingly, any nutrition intervention should be based on a thorough assessment of a patient's typical food intake and eating habits and should include an evaluation of current nutritional status.

Some patients with mild-to-moderate diabetes can be effectively treated with an appropriate balance of diet modification and exercise as the sole therapeutic intervention, particularly if their fasting blood glucose level is < 200 mg/dL. The majority of patients, however, will require pharmacologic intervention in addition to diet and exercise prescriptions. It is important to note that no pharmacologic treatment will be successful if the patient is not on some type of dietary and exercise regimen.

Dietary changes do not have to be dramatic to produce clinically important results in terms of lowering blood glucose and lipid levels. Regular monitoring of blood glucose, glycated hemoglobin, lipid levels, blood pressure, and body weight serves as an ongoing assessment of the nutrition intervention.

Nutrition Consult

Because nutrition issues and meal planning are complex, a registered dietitian who is familiar with the current principles and recommendations for managing diabetes may be consulted after a patient is diagnosed with diabetes. This health-care professional can be an essential member of the diabetes management team and performs valuable functions:

- Conducts initial assessment of nutritional status:
  - Diet history
  - Lifestyle
  - Eating habits
- Provides patient education regarding:
  - The basic principles of diet therapy for diabetes
  - Meal planning
  - Problem-solving techniques for changing eating behaviors
- Develops an individualized meal plan:
  - Emphasizing one or two priorities
  - Minimizing changes from the patient's usual diet (to encourage compliance)

- Provides follow-up assessment of the meal plan to:
  - Determine effectiveness in terms of glucose and lipid control and weight loss
  - Make necessary changes based on weight loss, activity level, or changes in medication
- Provides ongoing patient education and support (particularly for those on weight-loss regimens), helping patients learn to adjust their meal plans for various situations.

Body Weight Considerations 5

Weight loss frequently is a primary goal of nutrition therapy because 80% to 90% of people with type II diabetes are obese.[2] Caloric restriction and weight loss, even as small as 5% to 10% of body weight, can result in:
- Improved glucose control
- Increased sensitivity to insulin
- Lower lipid levels and blood pressure
- The need for a corresponding lowering of the dosage of pharmacologic agents (eg, oral hypoglycemic medications and insulin).

Weight loss is associated with improved glucose uptake and insulin sensitivity as well as decreased hepatic glucose production. Consequently, the therapeutic regimen most useful for individuals with obesity and glucose intolerance is weight reduction via nutrition therapy and increased physical activity. If moderate weight loss does not improve metabolic parameters, however, pharmacologic therapy (oral hypoglycemic agents or insulin) may need to be added to the regimen.

Weight loss and subsequent weight maintenance can be the most difficult and challenging aspect of managing diabetes. Therefore, emphasis should be

43

placed on achieving and maintaining normal blood glucose control as the goal of nutrition therapy, using nutritionally balanced meal plans that promote gradual weight loss as a means to achieve this metabolic goal. A reasonable approach that provides a combination of the following strategies increases the chances of a successful outcome:

- Modest caloric restriction
- Spreading caloric intake throughout the day
- Increased physical activity
- Behavior modification techniques for changing eating habits and attitudes and promoting healthy, long-term lifestyle behaviors
- Psychosocial support.

Suggested weights for adults based on the USDA *Dietary Guidelines for Americans* (1990) are shown in Table 5.1. The upper end of the ranges are considered appropriate weights for men, given their greater bone and muscle mass; the lower end of the ranges are for women, who have comparatively less bone and muscle mass.

Approximately 10% of patients with type II diabetes are of normal weight and do not need to modify their caloric intake. For these individuals, nutrition therapy focuses on distributing calorie and carbohydrate intake throughout the day to achieve optimal glucose control. The pattern of spreading out calories and carbohydrates between meals and snacks is individualized based on results of self-monitoring of blood glucose.

Calorie Intake

Adult calorie needs vary according to age, activity level, and desired weight change. The following procedure can be used to determine adult calorie requirements.[3] First calculate desired body weight:

44

Height	Weight (lb)	
	19 - 34 (yr)	≥ 35 (yr)
5' 0"	97-128	108-138
5' 1"	101-132	111-143
5' 2"	104-137	115-148
5' 3"	107-141	119-152
5' 4"	111-146	122-157
5' 5"	114-150	126-162
5' 6"	118-155	130-167
5' 7"	121-160	134-172
5' 8"	125-164	138-178
5' 9"	129-169	142-183
5'10"	132-174	146-188
5'11"	136-179	151-194
6' 0"	140-184	155-199
6' 1"	144-189	159-205
6' 2"	148-195	164-210
6' 3"	152-200	168-216
6' 4"	156-205	173-222
6' 5"	160-211	173-222
6' 6"	164-216	182-234

TABLE 5.1 — SUGGESTED WEIGHT FOR ADULTS

Source: US Department of Agriculture. US Department of Health and Human Services. *Nutrition and Your Health: Dietary Guidelines for Americans*, 3rd ed. Hyattsville, Md: USDA Human Nutrition Information Service; 1990.

- Women: 100 lb for the first 5 ft of height plus 5 lb for each additional inch over 5 ft
- Men: 106 lb for the first 5 ft of height plus 6 lb for each additional inch over 5 ft
- Add 10% for larger body builds; subtract 10% for smaller body builds.

Then, multiply the resulting weight by one of the following to compute calorie need based on desired weight:

- Men and physically active women: multiply by 15
- Most women, sedentary men, and adults over age 55: multiply by 13
- Sedentary women, obese adults, sedentary adults over age 55: multiply by 10.

If weight loss is indicated, daily calorie intake needs to be adjusted to produce the necessary deficit. Given that a 3500-calorie deficit per week is required to produce a 1-pound loss of fat, a decrease of approximately 500 to 1000 calories per day is needed to lose 1 to 2 pounds of fat per week. Regular exercise is an excellent way to create a calorie deficit and has been associated with successful weight maintenance. Because calorie restriction alone be difficult to maintain, some people have greater success by eliminating 250 to 500 calories from their daily diet and increasing daily activity by 250 to 500 calories.

Nutrient Composition of the Diet

A nutritionally balanced diet is as important for individuals with diabetes as for nondiabetics. Diet prescriptions for those with type II diabetes need to take into account the higher prevalence of hyperlipidemia, atherosclerosis, and hypertension in this population.

■ Protein Intake

The Recommended Dietary Allowance (RDA) for adults as advised by the USDA is used as the guideline for protein intake for patients with type II diabetes (0.8 g/kg body weight/day). This equates to a small-to-medium portion of protein once daily with either breakfast, lunch, or dinner. Protein allowance therefore amounts to 12% to 20% of daily calories and should be derived from both animal and vegetable sources. Vegetable protein may be less nephrotoxic than animal protein and thus restriction of vegetable protein may not be necessary. In following these recommendations, meat, fish, or poultry consumption would need to be limited to 3 to 5 oz daily.

Because excessive protein intake may aggravate renal insufficiency, type II patients with evidence of nephropathy should be encouraged to limit their protein intake to 12% of daily calories. In short-term studies, more severe restriction of protein (0.6 g/kg body weight/day) has been shown to be effective in slowing the progression of kidney disease in patients with diabetes who already have some renal insufficiency, but has been reported to be associated with loss of muscle mass and strength.[4-5] In addition, evidence exists that a low-protein diet can reverse the rate of deterioration in renal function.[5]

■ Fat Intake

The remaining 80% to 90% of daily calories are distributed between fat and carbohydrate intake, based on a patient's nutrition assessment and treatment goals (glucose, lipid, and weight outcomes). Several important benefits support the restriction of dietary fat in patients with type II diabetes:

- Excess consumption of dietary fat may contribute to obesity, which is common in the majority of patients with type II diabetes. Restricting dietary fat may limit the development or reduce the extent of obesity.

- Abnormal lipid levels often are associated with both obesity and diabetes and increase the risk of cardiovascular disease. Reduced intake of saturated fat can have beneficial effects by reducing triglyceride and low-density lipoprotein (LDL) cholesterol, and increasing high-density lipoprotein (HDL) cholesterol.

Therefore, the following guidelines are recommended for fat intake to promote weight loss, achieve lipid goals, and reduce cardiovascular risk:

- Reduce dietary fat to < 35% of total calories
- Limit saturated fat to < 10% of total calories, and < 7% of calories in patients with elevated LDL cholesterol
- Limit polyunsaturated fats to 10% of total calories
- Limit daily cholesterol consumption to 300 mg
- Moderately increase intake of monounsaturated fats such as canola and olive oil (up to 20% of calories). A diet high in monounsaturated fats has been shown to improve glucose control, lower triglycerides, and raise HDL levels.

Effectiveness of dietary fat modification is determined by regular monitoring of glycemic control, triglyceride and cholesterol status, and body weight, with periodic adjustments based on metabolic response to the diet.

■ Carbohydrate Intake

The carbohydrate allowance is determined after protein and fat intake have been calculated and is individualized based on eating habits and glucose and lipid goals. Emphasis is placed on whole grains, starches, fruits, and vegetables to provide the necessary vitamins, minerals, and fiber in the diet. The recommended daily consumption of fiber is the same for people with diabetes as for nondiabetics (20 g to 35 g). Although dietary fiber can improve serum lipid levels, the effect on glycemic control is minimal.

Traditionally, complex carbohydrates were thought to produce lower blood glucose responses than simple sugars because sugars are digested and absorbed more rapidly. This belief, which influenced previous recommendations of replacing simple sugars in the diet with complex carbohydrates, has been disproved by clinical research. For example, the glycemic response to fruits and milk has been found to be lower than the response to most starches, and sucrose has been found to produce a glycemic response similar to that of bread, rice, and potatoes.[6] The rate of digestion of a given food seems to be more related to the presence of fat, degree of ripeness, cooking method, and preparation.[1]

■ Sucrose

A modest amount of sugar is allowed in the daily diet of patients with type II diabetes. Sucrose and sucrose-containing foods may be substituted for other carbohydrates in the meal plan, but not simply added.[1,6] Patients need to be taught how to make such substitutions using self-monitoring of capillary blood glucose (SMCBG) to evaluate the glycemic response. The total nutrient content of the sucrose-containing food should be considered, particularly because sugar and fat are the main ingredients in many sweets. Obese individuals usually are advised to avoid sweets because of the potential of a small portion triggering overconsumption.

■ Fructose

A natural source of dietary fructose is fruits and vegetables. In addition, some sweeteners are derived from these sources. Moderate consumption is recommended, particularly concerning foods in which fructose is used as a sweetening agent. Although fructose has a lower glycemic effect than sucrose, it contains the same amount of calories and therefore should be limited in hypocaloric diets.[1] People with dyslipidemia also are advised to limit their consumption of fructose because of the potential adverse effects on serum triglyceride and LDL cholesterol levels.

■ Other Nutritive/Nonnutritive Sweeteners and Fat Substitutes

Nutritive sweeteners such as corn syrup, fruit juice/concentrate, honey, molasses, dextrose, and maltose do not seem to have a greater advantage or disadvantage over sucrose in terms of impact on calorie content or glycemic response, but they need to be accounted for in the meal plan.[1,6] Certain sugar alcohols (sorbitol, mannitol, xylitol) that commonly are used as sweeteners can produce a lower glycemic response than sucrose but seem to have no real advantage over sucrose or other nutritive sweeteners when consumed as part of mixed meals. Excessive consumption of sugar alcohols may cause laxative effects.

Nonnutritive sweeteners (saccharin, aspartame, acesulfame K) have been approved by the Food and Drug Administration (FDA) for consumption by people with diabetes.[6] These sweeteners are useful because they contribute no calories or carbohydrates to the diet when they are used as tabletop sweeteners or in soft drinks. However, when sweeteners are used in foods that contain other nutrients and calories (ice cream, cookies, puddings), the foods must be worked into the meal plan.[1]

Because many of the fat substitutes currently being used are derived from carbohydrate or protein sources, the content of these compounds is increased above the usual amounts in such products.[1] Patients need to be advised to review the carbohydrate and/or

protein content when using products with fat substitutes.

■ Vitamins and Minerals

Supplementation generally is not recommended
for people with diabetes when dietary intake is adequate and balanced. Patients who become chromium-
deficient as a result of long-term parenteral nutrition
may require chromium supplementation.[6] However,
most people with diabetes are not chromium-deficient
and do not benefit from supplementation. Similarly,
magnesium does not need to be added to the diets of
most patients with diabetes unless routine evaluation
of serum magnesium reveals a deficiency. Patients
taking diuretics may need potassium supplementation.
However, hyperkalemia may require potassium restriction in patients with renal insufficiency, or hyporeninemic hypoaldosteronism, or in those taking angiotensin-converting enzyme (ACE) inhibitors.[6] One
consideration may be the potential value of antioxidant supplements (vitamins E, C, and beta-carotene)
in reducing atherosclerotic lesions and cataracts, both
of which are common in type II diabetes. The value
of such supplementation is yet to be confirmed.

■ Alcohol Intake

The same recommendations used for the general
population are appropriate for people with type II diabetes. Moderate consumption will not adversely affect blood glucose in patients whose diabetes is well
controlled. Calories from alcohol should be included
as part of the total calorie intake and reflected in the
meal plan as a substitute for fat (one alcoholic beverage = two fat exchanges). For patients taking insulin,
one or two alcoholic beverages per day are acceptable
(one alcoholic beverage = 12 oz beer, 5 oz wine, or
1½ oz distilled spirits; sweet drinks should be avoided)
taken with or in addition to the meal plan. However,

some special considerations exist regarding alcohol intake. Patients taking insulin or sulfonylureas are susceptible to hypoglycemia if alcohol is consumed on an empty stomach. Therefore, these individuals should make sure to take any desired alcohol with a meal. Patients with diabetes and coexisting medical problems such as pancreatitis, dyslipidemis, or neuropathy may need to reduce or abstain from alcohol intake.

REFERENCES

1. American Diabetes Association. *Medical Management of Non–insulin-dependent (Type II) Diabetes,* 3rd ed. Alexandria, Va: American Diabetes Association; 1994:22-39.

2. American Diabetes Association. *Diabetes 1996 Vital Statistics*. Alexandria, Va: American Diabetes Association; 1996.

3. Davidson MB. *Diabetes Mellitus*: *Diagnosis and Treatment*, 3rd ed. New York: Churchill Livingstone; 1991:35-93.

4. Henry RR. Protein content of the diabetic diet. *Diabetes Care*. 1994;17:1502-1513.

5. Mudaliar SR, Henry RR. Role of glycemic control and protein restriction in clinical management of diabetic kidney disease. *Endocr Pract*. 1996;2:220-226.

6. American Diabetes Association. Clinical practice recommendations 1995. Position statement: nutrition recommendations and principles for people with diabetes mellitus. *Diabetes Care*. 1995;18(suppl 1):16-19.

6   Exercise

Many adults with diabetes are sedentary as a result of their obesity, which can contribute to the development of glucose intolerance. Therefore, physical activity should be included as an essential treatment component in the diabetes management plan unless contraindicated in a given individual. Current research even suggests that regular exercise can prevent or delay the onset of type II diabetes in susceptible, high-risk individuals.

Benefits

The potential benefits of regular exercise include:[1]
- Improved glucose tolerance because of enhanced insulin sensitivity
- Weight loss or maintenance of a desirable body weight because of increased energy expenditure
- Improved cardiovascular risk factors
- Improved response to pharmacologic therapy, with the potential of reducing the dosage or the need for insulin or oral hypoglycemic agents
- Improved energy level, muscular strength, flexibility, quality of life, and sense of well-being.

Precautions and Considerations

Because many people with diabetes have not been active and are deconditioned, exercise should be started at a low level and gradually increased to avoid adverse effects such as injury, hypoglycemia, or cardiac problems. Most adults with diabetes should have a physical examination, including a stress test, before beginning to exercise to rule out significant cardiovascular disease or silent ischemia and determine the presence of any diabetic complications. Strenuous activity is not recommended for patients with poor metabolic control and those with significant complications.

Patients being treated with sulfonylureas or insulin are susceptible to hypoglycemia during or as much as 12 hours after exercising.[1] To prevent hypoglycemia, these patients should use self-monitoring of capillary blood glucose (SMCBG) both before and after exercising to determine their response to varying degrees of physical activity. Appropriate consumption of snacks as needed can help avert most problems. More importantly, establishing and following a regular exercise program can reduce the likelihood of exercise-induced episodes of hypoglycemia.

Exercise Prescription

Any exercise prescription should be individualized to account for patient interests, physical status and capacity, and motivation. Although having a planned program of physical activity is ideal, exercise is so important and beneficial that just getting patients moving is a worthwhile initial goal. Patients should choose activities that are appropriate for their general physical condition and lifestyle, start slowly, and work up to the goal of performing an aerobic activity at 50% to 70% of maximum oxygen uptake at least 3 to 4 times per week, with a minimum duration of 20 minutes per session (ideally 30 to 40 minutes).[1-2] Weight reduction is enhanced by exercising 5 to 6 times per week. Recommended aerobic activities include:

- Walking
- Biking and stationary cycling
- Lap swimming and aerobic water exercises.

Muscle-strengthening exercises such as lifting light weights also should be included in an exercise program, as well as flexibility stretches during warm-ups and cool-downs.

Guidelines for safe exercise should be reviewed with patients (Table 6.1).

TABLE 6.1 — GENERAL EXERCISE GUIDELINES

- Exercise stress test should be performed in most adults with diabetes to rule out significant cardiovascular disease or silent ischemia.

- Start slowly at a low level; gradually increase intensity and frequency.

- Carry identification including diabetes medical identification.

- Monitor blood glucose preexercise and postexercise.

- Be alert for signs of hypoglycemia during and several hours after exercising; carry appropriate carbohydrate source if necessary.

- Closely monitor blood glucose when exercise intensity is increased.

- Drink sufficient fluids before, during, and after exercise to maintain adequate hydration.

REFERENCES

1. American Diabetes Association. *Medical Management of Non–insulin-dependent (Type II) Diabetes,* 3rd ed. Alexandria, Va: American Diabetes Association; 1994:22-39.

2. American Diabetes Association. Clinical practice recommendations 1995. Position statement: diabetes mellitus and exercise. *Diabetes Care*. 1995;18(suppl 1):28.

7   Oral Agents

The majority of patients with type II diabetes have less than ideal metabolic control despite our greater understanding of the underlying pathophysiologic mechanisms of hyperglycemia and the availability of a wide variety of treatment options. Failure to achieve glycemic goals is related in part to a misconception by patients and caregivers that type II diabetes is a mild disease, and not as serious as type I diabetes. In fact, type II diabetes in many respects may be a more deadly disease than type I diabetes because of the multiple cardiovascular risk factors associated with this form of diabetes.

Hyperglycemia in type II diabetes often coexists with several other metabolic abnormalities such as obesity, hypertension, dyslipidemia, and accelerated atherosclerosis, which themselves require prompt and aggressive diagnosis and treatment. Moreover, prolonged hyperglycemia leads to a worsening of the insulin resistance and endogenous insulin secretory ability (glucose toxicity), thus contributing to the primary and secondary oral agent failure rate. Aggressive management to reduce the hyperglycemia, which in many cases may require temporary insulin therapy, is necessary to reverse the glucose toxic state.

Pharmacologic therapy with oral antidiabetic agents is required when dietary modification and exercise therapy do not result in normalization or near normalization of metabolic abnormalities. Pharmacologic therapy should always be considered as adjunctive therapy to diet and exercise, and not as a substitute. Although maintaining an ideal diet and exercise regimen is difficult, it is important to emphasize that no

pharmacologic therapy can be expected to be successful if the patient is not following some type of dietary
and exercise program.

Pathophysiologic Basis of Pharmacologic Therapy

The treatment strategies selected for managing type
II diabetes are based on an understanding of the pathophysiology of hyperglycemia and the unique clinical
expression of the associated metabolic abnormalities
in an individual. Type II diabetes is characterized by
three basic abnormalities that contribute to the development of hyperglycemia:

- Excessive glucose production by the liver
- Impaired insulin secretion by the pancreas
- Peripheral insulin resistance mainly in the skel-
  etal muscle.

Fasting and postprandial hyperglycemia varies
considerably among individuals depending upon the
extent, severity, and unique expression of each of these
metabolic abnormalities, and these differences also play
a role in the various responses to the different classes
of oral antidiabetic agents. Such differences are exem-
plified by the lean and obese varieties of type II diabetes, which exhibit the same underlying pathophysiology but differ in the extent to which each abnormality
contributes to the development of the hyperglycemic
state. In lean, type II diabetic patients, impaired insulin
secretion is the predominant defect, while insulin resistance tends to be less severe than in the obese variety. Insulin resistance and hyperinsulinemia are the
classic abnormalities of obese individuals with type II
diabetes. In general, the oral antidiabetic agents are
most effective early in the course of diabetes when
insulin deficiency is not the predominant abnormality.

Intensive Therapy in Type II Diabetes

Two long-term studies of intensive diabetes management in type I diabetes provide clear-cut evidence that near-normalization of glycemia can prevent and delay the development and progression of retinopathy, nephropathy, and neuropathy in type I diabetes.[1-2] Patients with type II diabetes are also likely to receive comparable benefits from an intensive therapeutic approach to control glycemia because the severity and duration of hyperglycemia has a critical role in the development and progression of microvascular complications, regardless of the etiology of the hyperglycemia. There are now studies that demonstrate not only a reduction in microvascular disease in type II diabetes with improved glycemic control, but also reductions in dyslipidemia and coronary artery disease. In addition, there are no published reports demonstrating any serious adverse effects of near normalization of the glucose values in type II diabetes other than weight gain and hypoglycemia. Thus, similar intensive management strategies, including all facets of diabetes care that are applied rigorously to achieve normal or near-normal glycemia, are warranted for patients with type II diabetes and should be attempted whenever possible.

The American Diabetes Association[3] has responded to the implications of these preventative studies by revising its therapeutic glycemic goals to advocate tighter metabolic control in type I and type II diabetes (Table 7.1). Intensive therapy with diet, exercise, and antidiabetic agents may be the most effective way to achieve these goals in patients with type II diabetes.

Oral Antidiabetic Agents

Oral medication is initiated when 3 months of diet and exercise alone are unable to achieve or maintain plasma glucose levels within these glycemic guidelines.

TABLE 7.1 — CURRENT ADA GLYCEMIC GUIDELINES			
Biochemical Index	**Normal**	**Goal**	**Action Suggested**
Fasting/preprandial glucose	< 115 mg/dL (< 6.4 mM)	< 120 mg/dL (< 6.7 mM)	< 80 or > 140 mg/dL (< 4.4 or > 7.8 mM)
Bedtime glucose	< 120 mg/dL (< 6.7 mM)	100-140 mg/dL (5.6-7.8 mM)	< 100 or > 160 mg/dL (< 5.6 or > 8.9 mM)
Glycated hemoglobin*	< 6%	< 7%	> 8%

* Referenced to a nondiabetic range of 4% to 6% (mean 5%, SD 0.5%).

Source: American Diabetes Association. *Medical Management of Non–insulin-dependent (Type II) Diabetes*, 3rd ed. Alexandria, Va: American Diabetes Association; 1994:26.

Current therapy for the treatment of hyperglycemia of type II diabetes includes the following oral antidiabetic agents:

- First- and second-generation sulfonylureas
- The biguanide metformin
- The alpha-glucosidase inhibitor acarbose.

Until recently (before the availability of metformin and acarbose in the United States), approximately 35% of type II patients were treated with insulin. In Europe, the number of insulin-requiring type II diabetics is approximately 10% lower because of the availability of these new oral agents. In the United States, nearly 64% of adults with type II diabetes use oral therapy during the first 5 years after diagnosis; this figure drops to 37% after a 20-year duration of diabetes. The explanation for this secondary failure rate is that as time goes on, the endogenous insulin secretory ability of the pancreas diminishes and the need for exogenous insulin increases. It is believed that by intensifying glycemic control early, one can possibly delay this consistently observed beta cell exhaustion phenomenon.

Oral antidiabetic agents have different pharmacokinetics, potency, metabolism, and other factors that influence the choice of medication to use for initial and combination therapy (Table 7.2). In general, oral agents are contraindicated in patients who:

- Are pregnant or lactating
- Are seriously ill
- Have significant kidney or liver disease
- Have demonstrated allergic reactions.

In addition, patients with significant and prolonged hyperglycemia with marked symptoms such as weight loss should be considered for temporary insulin therapy before considering the institution of oral agents.

TABLE 7.2 — CHARACTERISTICS OF CURRENTLY AVAILABLE ORAL ANTIDIABETIC AGENTS*

Generic Name	Trade Name	Recommended Starting Dosage, mg†	Recommended Maximum Dosage, mg	Duration of Action, h
SULFONYLUREAS				
First Generation				
Acetohexamide	Dymelor	125 bid	750 bid	10-14
Chlorpropamide	Diabinese	250 qd	500 qd	60
Tolazamide	Tolinase	100 qd	500 bid	12-24
Tolbutamide	Orinase	250 bid	1000 tid	6-12
Second Generation				
Glimepiride	Amaryl	1-2 qd	8 qd	24
Glipizide	Glucotrol	5 qd	20 bid	12-24
Glipizide (extended release)	Glucotrol XL	5 qd	20 qd	24
Glyburide	DiaBeta, Micronase	2.5-5 qd	10 bid	16-24
	Glynase PresTab	1.5-3 qd	6 bid	12-24

BIGUANIDE			
Metformin	Glucophage	500 bid‡	2500	Plasma elimination half-life is ~6.2
ALPHA-GLUCOSIDASE INHIBITOR			
Acarbose	Precose	25 tid‡	100 tid	Not absorbed systemically

* See section on new oral drugs in development.

† Starting dosage for elderly and lean adults with diabetes may need to be reduced by 50%.

‡ The dosage of metformin and acarbose must be titrated slowly.

Source: *Physicians' Desk Reference*, 51st ed. Montvale, NJ: Medical Economics Data Production Company; 1997.

7

Sulfonylureas

Sulfonylureas work primarily by stimulating pancreatic insulin secretion, which in turn reduces hepatic glucose output and increases peripheral glucose disposal.

Four first-generation sulfonylurea compounds have been available in the United States for the treatment of type II diabetes for over 20 years. They are:
- Acetohexamide
- Chlorpropamide
- Tolazamide
- Tolbutamide.

Two second-generation sulfonylurea compounds (glipizide and glyburide) were introduced in the United States in 1984 and another (glimepiride) more recently. Thus, the second-generation compounds are:
- Glimepiride
- Glipizide
- Glyburide.

The efficacy of the first- and second-generation sulfonylureas is similar, although second-generation agents are better formulated and have some advantages. Second-generation sulfonylureas:
- Are more potent on a per milligram basis
- Tend to produce fewer side effects
- Interact less frequently with other drugs.

Improved formulations of glipizide (Glucotrol XL) and glyburide (Glynase PresTab) are also available. In addition, the pharmacokinetics of these second-generation agents allows for more effective once-a-day dosing, which enhances compliance.

■ Side Effects of Sulfonylureas

Most of the side effects associated with sulfonylurea therapy are mild, infrequent, and occur less often with the second-generation agents; they include:

- Mild gastrointestinal upset
- Skin reactions
  - Rashes
  - Purpura
  - Pruritus
- Weight gain (this effect can be minimized or prevented by increasing emphasis on dietary habits).

Hyponatremia, fluid retention, and the Antabuse reaction have also been reported with the use of chlorpropamide. The major complication of sulfonylurea therapy is severe hypoglycemia, which has been more of a problem with chlorpropamide than with any other agent because of its long half-life and duration of action. Hypoglycemia also is more common in individuals who consume large amounts of alcohol and skip meals. Glipizide is reported to have a lower risk of hypoglycemia because it is metabolized to inactive by-products that do not have hypoglycemic activity. Other reactions are rare and include:

- Hematologic reactions
  - Leukopenia
  - Thrombocytopenia
  - Hemolytic anemia
- Cholestasis (with and without jaundice).

■ Prescribing Sulfonylureas

In general, therapy should be initiated at the lowest possible dose, especially in the elderly (Table 7.2). It is begun once daily, before breakfast, and increased progressively every 1 to 2 weeks until the desired therapeutic glycemic response is achieved or the maximum dose is reached. The dosing regimen is changed to twice daily when the daily dose approaches 50% or more of the maximum recommended dose. Dosing adjustments can also be made based on self-monitoring of capillary blood glucose (SMCBG) data. For example, if the patient's SMCBG results show elevated fasting blood glucose values, then the evening dose should be titrated upward. If, on the other hand, the evening blood glucose values are elevated, then the morning dose can be raised.

Clinicians should focus on achieving satisfactory glycemic control and not concentrate solely on the patient's symptoms, which could lead to premature dosage discontinuation or reduction. In patients with glucose toxicity and markedly elevated glucose values (ie, > 200-300 mg/dL), it may be possible to achieve successful treatment by starting with a maximum dose of a sulfonylurea and tapering the dose later, as the glucose values fall. These patients need close monitoring and should have SMCBG equipment available. Patients who do not achieve appropriate glycemic control in response to an adequate trial of maximum doses of a sulfonylurea may respond to combination therapy with other oral agents and/or insulin therapy.

■ First-generation Sulfonylureas

Acetohexamide

Acetohexamide (Dymelor) is rapidly absorbed, has an intermediate duration of action, and demonstrates maximum hypoglycemic activity within 3 hours. In persons with normal renal and hepatic function, more than 80% of the drug is excreted in 24 hours. Recommended dosing is twice daily.

Chlorpropamide

Chlorpropamide (Diabinese) is rapidly absorbed and partially metabolized by the liver to products that retain hypoglycemic activity, thus explaining the long duration of action (60 hrs). Approximately 70% of the drug is metabolized and about 30% is excreted intact in the urine. Recommended dosing is once daily. Chlorpropamide can cause prolonged hypoglycemia, significant hyponatremia, and a mild Antabuse-like reaction (flushing and headache with alcohol consumption) in some patients. Elderly patients are more susceptible to hypoglycemia, particularly if they have impaired renal function or tend to skip meals. For these reasons, this drug generally is not recommended for elderly patients.

Tolazamide

Tolazamide (Tolinase) is absorbed slowly, demonstrates hypoglycemic effects within 4 to 6 hours, and has an intermediate duration of action. It is metabolized by the liver to by-products with little hypoglycemic activity that are excreted in the urine. Most patients require a second daily dose.

Tolbutamide

Tolbutamide (Orinase) is a short-acting sulfonylurea with a rapid onset of action and peak concentration within 2 to 3 hours. It is metabolized by the liver to inactive products, most of which are excreted in the urine within 24 hours. Recommended dosing is 2 to 3 times daily because of its short half-life.

■ Second-generation Sulfonylureas

Glimepiride

Glimepiride (Amaryl) is a new sulfonylurea agent recently approved by the Food and Drug Administration (FDA). Amaryl therapy has been shown to improve overall glucose control without producing clinically meaningful increases in fasting and C-peptide levels. It is the only sulfonylurea with an FDA-approved indication for combination therapy with insulin.

The usual maintenance dosage is 1 mg to 4 mg once daily. The maximum recommended dosage is 8 mg once daily. After reaching a dose of 2 mg, dosage increases should be made in increments of no more than 2 mg at 1 to 2 week intervals based on the patient's blood glucose response.

Glipizide

Glipizide (Glucotrol, Glucotrol XL) is a second-generation sulfonylurea that is metabolized by the liver to inactive products, reducing the risk of hypoglycemia. Glucotrol XL utilizes a controlled delivery system, and when compared with the immediate-release Glucotrol, the risk of hypoglycemia and the glucose and insulin responses to meals are similar although compliance is improved. Glipizide is particularly suited for the elderly or any patient with mild renal or liver dysfunction. Recommended dosing is normally 1 to 2 times daily for immediate-release glipizide. The long-acting extended-release formulation (Glucotrol XL) maintains therapeutic plasma levels effectively for 24 hours, and once-daily dosing is adequate in the majority of patients.

Glyburide

Glyburide (DiaBeta, Micronase, Glynase PresTab) is metabolized by the liver to mostly inert products that are excreted in the urine and bile. However, some of the by-products do have hypoglycemic activity and caution is advised, especially in patients with evidence of liver or kidney dysfunction. The duration of action is 16 to 24 hours, and recommended dosing is 1 to 2 times daily. A micronized particle formulation facilitates rapid absorption (Glynase PresTab).

■ Drug Interactions With Sulfonylureas

A number of drugs can interfere with the hypoglycemic action of sulfonylurea drugs, and some can alter the effects of sulfonylureas (Table 7.3). Co-administration of these drugs with sulfonylureas must be monitored closely.

TABLE 7.3 — DRUGS THAT POTENTIATE THE HYPOGLYCEMIC EFFECTS OF THE SULFONYLUREA AGENTS

Generic Name	Trade Name(s)
Sulfonamides	
Sulfacytine	Renoquid
Sulfadiazine	Microsulfon
Sulfamethoxazole	Azo Gantanol,* Bactrim* Gantanol, Septra,* Urobak
Sulfamethizole	Thiosulfil, Proklar,* Urobiotic*
Sulfisoxazole	Azo Gantrisin,* Eryzole* Gantrisin, Pediazole,* SK-Soxazole*
Chloramphenicol	Chloromycetin
Bishydroxycoumarin	Dicumarol
Phenylbutazone	Butazolidin
Oxyphenbutazone	Tandearil
Clofibrate	Atromid-S
* Combination drug.	

Source: American Diabetes Association. *Medical Management of Non–insulin-dependent (Type II) Diabetes*, 3rd ed. Alexandria, Va: American Diabetes Association; 1994:40-49.

Metformin

Metformin (Glucophage) is a biguanide that works mainly by:

- Suppressing excessive hepatic glucose production
- Increasing glucose utilization in peripheral tissues.

Metformin may also improve glucose levels by reducing intestinal glucose absorption. Because metformin does not stimulate endogenous insulin secretion, hypoglycemia does not occur when this dose is used alone, although hypoglycemia may occur if metformin is taken with insulin, a sulfonylurea, or an excessive amount of alcohol. Metformin is not metabolized and is excreted unchanged by the kidneys.

Metformin is effective as monotherapy or in combination with sulfonylureas, alpha-glucosidase inhibitors, and insulin. Metformin can be added to the regimens of patients who have not responded initially to sulfonylureas (primary treatment failure) or patients who responded initially to sulfonylureas, but who subsequently have deterioration of glycemic control (secondary treatment failure).[4] Sulfonylureas can also be added to the regimens of patients failing metformin therapy. The combination of metformin and a sulfonylurea often achieves a better glycemic response than either agent given alone.[4]

Treatment with metformin has additional beneficial effects on plasma lipids (it lowers triglyceride and low-density lipoprotein [LDL] cholesterol levels while increasing high-density lipoprotein [HDL] cholesterol), that are greater than the expected improvement in the lipid profile seen with better glucose control. In addition, metformin therapy has been associated with weight loss or no weight gain. This may be particularly helpful in obese patients with type II diabetes.

■ Side Effects of Metformin

The major side effects of metformin are:
- Gastrointestinal effects, consisting mainly of mild diarrhea
- Anorexia
- Nausea
- Abdominal discomfort.

For most patients, these side effects:
- Are transient
- Are dose related
- Tend to decrease with chronic therapy.

They can be minimized by:
- Slow dosage titration
- Decreasing the dosage
- Taking metformin with meals.

Lactic acidosis is a rare complication of metformin therapy and has a high mortality rate. Most of the cases of metformin-associated lactic acidosis occurred in patients for whom the drug was contraindicated, ie, patients with renal dysfunction. Metformin should not be prescribed if the serum creatinine is greater than 1.5 mg/dL in men or greater than 1.4 mg/dL in women. Metformin is also contraindicated in patients with significant hepatic disease, cardiac insufficiency, alcohol abuse, and any hypoxic condition or history of lactic acidosis. Metformin should be temporarily discontinued 1 to 2 days before any dye studies so that serum metformin levels are low if the patient develops renal failure from the dye. In any patient who is hospitalized with an acute severe illness, metformin should be temporarily discontinued.

■ **Prescribing Metformin**
Suggested initial dosing is 500 mg/day with dinner for 1 week, then twice daily with breakfast and dinner. The dosage should be titrated slowly, as needed, toward a maximum daily dose of 2500 mg. A third dose can be safely added at bedtime instead of at noon. The compliance is better and metformin at bedtime works well to suppress hepatic glucose production at night. Several weeks are required to see the maximum effect of metformin once a stable dosage is achieved.

Acarbose

Acarbose (Precose) is an alpha-glucosidase inhibitor that slows down the breakdown of disaccharides and polysaccharides and other complex carbohydrates into monosaccharides. The enzymatic generation and subsequent absorption of glucose is delayed and the postprandial blood glucose values, which are characteristically high in patients with type II diabetes, are reduced. The postprandial blood glucose has been an overlooked value and can significantly contribute to prolonged hyperglycemia. Acarbose is an excellent pharmacologic agent to "spread the calories" which is recommended by the American Diabetes Association and has been shown to smooth out daytime glycemia.

Acarbose has proven to be an effective agent when used alone or in combination with other antidiabetic agents. Acarbose has been shown to reduce the postprandial glucose value by at least 50 mg/dL and the fasting glucose by 10 to 20 mg/dL. Acarbose also lowers the postprandial integrated insulin levels, as less glucose is being presented to the pancreas at any one time. Acarbose does not stimulate insulin release and does not cause hypoglycemia when used alone. The average reduction in glycosylated hemoglobin is usually 0.7% to 1.0%. Since acarbose reduces the postprandial blood glucose and does not cause hypoglycemia, the drop in $HgbA_{1C}$ is not as dramatic as one would see with the sulfonylureas which can cause hypoglycemia (the $HgbA_{1C}$ is an average of the highs and lows). Although the combined use of acarbose with metformin and/or insulin has not yet received official approval by the FDA, acarbose has been used successfully with all other oral agents and insulin for the treatment of type II diabetes.[5]

■ **Side Effects of Acarbose**

The main side effect of acarbose is flatulence. Soft stools or diarrhea and mild abdominal pain have also been reported. Many of the symptoms are dose related and transient, occurring with the highest frequency during the first 8 weeks of therapy. The symptoms are probably caused by the osmotic effect of undigested carbohydrates in the distal bowel. The most important factor in avoiding side effects is to titrate acarbose very slowly. Because acarbose is not absorbed systemically and does not cause hypoglycemia, it has been suggested that it may be safer than other oral agents in patients with kidney disease, in the elderly, and in children with type II diabetes.

■ **Prescribing Acarbose**

The recommended maintenance dosage of acarbose is 50 mg to 100 mg orally 3 times a day with meals. The suggested starting dosage of acarbose is 25 mg/day and should be titrated up slowly to the maintenance dosage of 50 mg to 100 mg tid to avoid side effects (see Table 7.4).

Monotherapy With Oral Antidiabetic Agents

The choice of therapy has become more complicated as a result of the availability of three different classes of oral antidiabetic agents. Patients should be evaluated on an individual basis considering these variables:

- Age
- Weight
- Duration of diabetes
- Presence of dyslipidemia
- Severity of hyperglycemia
- Presence of glucose toxicity

TABLE 7.4 — PRECOSE™ (ACARBOSE) DOSING INSTRUCTIONS FOR PATIENTS

1. You have been given Precose because your blood sugar control needs to be improved. Precose is a very safe medication that has been proven effective in improving overall blood sugar control in people with diabetes.

2. Precose works by delaying the absorption of glucose in the gut or delaying the digestion of carbohydrates and subsequent absorption of glucose.

3. Precose reduces the rise in blood sugar that typically occurs after eating. Marked elevation in blood sugar after eating is a common yet important problem that often is overlooked.

4. Precose *may* cause flatulence (excess gas), mild stomach pain, and/or diarrhea. These side effects tend to occur at the beginning of therapy and can be lessened by starting with a low dose of Precose and increasing the dose very slowly.

5. Suggested dosing schedule:
   Step 1: Start with 25 mg* at breakfast only for 1 week
   Step 2: Take 25 mg with breakfast and dinner for 1 week
   Step 3: Take 25 mg with breakfast, lunch, and dinner for 1 week
   Step 4: Take 50 mg with breakfast and 25 mg with lunch and dinner for 1 week
   Step 5: Take 50 mg with breakfast and dinner, and 25 mg with lunch for 1 week
   Step 6: Take 50 mg with breakfast, lunch, and dinner[†]

6. Do not go to a higher step if you are having bothersome flatulence, stomach pain, or diarrhea. Stay at the current step or go to a lower step until your symptoms improve.

7. It is extremely important to take Precose with the beginning of your meal. Precose will not work to lower your blood sugar if you take it more than 10 minutes before you eat.

8. Do not hesitate to call Bayer, the manufacturer of Precose, if you have any questions or concerns. The patient information hotline number is 1-800-PRECOSE.

---

* Break the 50-mg pill in half or use a pill cutter.
† Do not increase your dose to 100 mg 3 times daily until you talk with your caregiver.

- Presence and degree of kidney and liver disease
- Presence of ulcer disease and other gastrointestinal problems.

In general, the traditional approach to patients with type II diabetes failing a nonpharmacologic approach is to start a sulfonylurea agent, although there may be certain clinical situations that warrant a different approach. Recommendations for several of the commonly seen clinical presentations of patients with type II diabetes are described below.

■ Obese Patients With Newly Diagnosed Diabetes With/Without Dyslipidemia

Metformin or acarbose has the advantage of not inducing weight gain, which can occur with sulfonylureas and insulin therapy. Either of these drugs is a good choice after an unsuccessful 3-month trial of nonpharmacologic intervention. The risk of hypoglycemia also is low because metformin and acarbose do not stimulate insulin secretion. Additional benefits of metformin include lowering of triglyceride levels and raising of HDL cholesterol. These effects are in addition to those resulting from improved glycemic control. Sulfonylurea agents are also effective as first-line therapy in this patient group, especially in patients whose fasting blood glucose levels are excessively high (> 250 mg/dL). Sulfonylureas are advantageous as they can be started at relatively high doses without the need for titrating because of the absence of gastrointestinal side effects.

■ Thin Elderly Patients

Thin patients in general do not respond well to oral agents. Caution should be used when prescribing any medication in the elderly, and starting doses need to be lower than those in younger patients. Metformin can be effective in all age groups, although caution should be used in elderly patients who are thin and have reduced muscle mass. Such individuals may have a serum creatinine level that is within the dosing guidelines (males < 1.5 mg/dL; females < 1.4 mg/dL), but may have reduced renal function. Creatinine clearance should be measured and metformin avoided when the creatinine clearance is less than 60 mL/min. A low-dose sulfonylurea may be effective, although the risk of hypoglycemia is higher in this population as they are more insulin sensitive because of their nonobese status. Glipizide would be a good choice in such patients because the metabolites do not have any hypoglycemic activity. Acarbose also represents a safe approach because:

- Its excretion is not dependent on renal function
- It is not absorbed systemically
- It does not cause hypoglycemia.

■ **Patients With Acceptable Fasting Glucose Values but Elevated Glycohemoglobin Levels**

This scenario suggests the likelihood of elevated postprandial glucose levels, which can be confirmed by SMCBG 1 to 2 hours after eating. An alpha-glucosidase inhibitor such as acarbose would be an appropriate choice in these patients because acarbose works mainly by reducing the postprandial glucose value. If acarbose is not indicated or tolerated, then a clinical trial of a sulfonylurea or metformin may be effective.

■ **Nonobese Individuals With Diabetes**

As mentioned earlier, thin patients usually do not respond as well to oral agents as do obese patients. Lean patients with mild glucose intolerance can be given a trial with any of the three classes of oral agents. A sulfonylurea or metformin may be a better choice for patients whose blood glucose values are consistently in the 200s to 300s, because these drugs can be titrated more rapidly to higher doses, which may be necessary in this patient group. Late onset type I diabetes should be considered in thin, older adults and is thought to occur in as many as 15% of "insulin-requiring type II diabetics," usually misdiagnosed as having type II diabetes because of their age. Because weeks to months can be wasted on unsuccessful trials of the various oral agents in this patient group, a fasting or meal-stimulated insulin or C-peptide level is a simple method to assure the correct diagnosis and better direct treatment strategies (ie, insulin therapy).

■ **Patients With Prolonged, Severe Hyperglycemia (Glucose Toxicity)**

Ideally, a temporary trial of insulin therapy should be instituted for a few weeks before beginning an oral agent to reduce insulin resistance and improve endogenous insulin secretory capacity (see Chapter 8, *Insulin Therapy*). Improvement of metabolic control will increase the likelihood of a successful trial with an oral agent. Starting an oral agent when a patient has had prolonged and severe hyperglycemia is one of the most common causes of primary failure with an oral agent. Another approach that has been used with some success is to start a sulfonylurea agent at the maximum dose and follow the patient carefully, usually with a SMCBG device. Once metabolic control is achieved with either insulin or maximum-dose sulfonylureas, the dosage requirements may fall as the glucose toxic state improves. Patients will have a greater chance of success if they remain on a calorie-restricted diet simultaneously.

■ **Patients With Severe Renal or Liver Dysfunction**

Both sulfonylureas and metformin should be used with caution in patients with renal or liver disease (depending on the extent of organ dysfunction). Patients with mild to moderate glucose intolerance can be treated with acarbose, although if the patient is symptomatic, insulin may need to be instituted.

Combination Therapy With Oral Antidiabetic Agents

Many patients with type II diabetes will not have adequate glycemic control with monotherapy. The reason a patient fails monotherapy is multifactorial, although the most common explanation is beta cell exhaustion, which reduces the response to oral agents. Combination therapy with two or more of the oral antidiabetic agents has been used extensively in many countries with excellent results. Each of the different combinations has certain advantages and disadvantages for any given patient. The various combinations are discussed below. In general, when monotherapy is failing, addition rather than substitution of another oral agent is usually required to improve metabolic control.

■ **Sulfonylureas and Metformin**
Sulfonylureas and metformin have been proven to be a very effective combination.[6] Patients failing maximum doses of either metformin or a sulfonylurea can be given the other medication in combination therapy. Some patients may have blood glucose values that are too low (ie, < 80 mg/dL) during the daytime after beginning combination therapy. In such cases, the sulfonylurea dose should be lowered to achieve consistent daytime glucose values in a safe range. Metformin will also blunt the weight gain that may occur with the use of sulfonylureas alone. The combination of a sulfonylurea and metformin tends to be more potent in terms of lowering glycosylated hemoglobin than any other two oral agents used together.

■ **Sulfonylureas and Acarbose**

Acarbose and sulfonylureas also work well together.[7] Acarbose, in a fashion similar to metformin, tends to blunt the weight gain that can occur with the sulfonylureas when they are used alone. Because of their unique mechanisms of action, acarbose and the sulfonylureas complement one another and can reduce both fasting and postprandial glucose values.

■ **Metformin and Acarbose**

Neither of these drugs causes weight gain or hypoglycemia when used alone or in combination. Metformin significantly affects the fasting blood glucose values, whereas acarbose primarily reduces the postprandial values. These two medications have been used together successfully without excessive gastrointestinal side effects.[5] Clinical trials are currently underway to determine the efficacy and safety of these agents in various combinations.

■ **Sulfonylureas, Metformin, and Acarbose**

In Europe, the combination of all three oral agents has been used in clinical practice. Each of these oral agents has a unique mechanism of action, and they can potentially complement each other to:
- Improve glycemic control in patients
- Avoid insulin therapy.

The cost effectiveness, safety, and efficacy of such a regimen have not been determined.

"Insulin Sensitizers"

A new class of investigational antidiabetic agents will soon be available for the treatment of type II diabetes. One such product is troglitazone, a compound from the thiazolidinedione class of drugs that reduces insulin resistance in diabetic and nondiabetic obese patients. It appears to exert direct effects to improve insulin action mainly in liver and skeletal muscle. Troglitazone improves glucose uptake in skeletal muscle and decreases glucose production by the liver. As a result, there is an improvement in both fasting and postprandial hyperglycemia in obese type II diabetes patients, with a near normalization of the elevated rates of hepatic glucose production. Reductions in fasting and postprandial insulinemia also result from troglitazone therapy. Troglitazone significantly lowers very low-density lipoprotein (VLDL) cholesterol, increases HDL cholesterol, and reduces blood pressure. Recent evidence indicates that troglitazone may also prevent patients with impaired glucose tolerance (IGT) from progressing to frank type II diabetes.[8] Other advantages of troglitazone include:

- Once-a-day dosing
- Lack of dependence on renal function for clearance
- Low side effect profile
- Antioxidant properties.

Taking Patients With Type II Diabetes Off Insulin

The availability of the new oral antidiabetic agents allows patients with type II diabetes to possibly be taken off insulin. This therapeutic strategy has not been studied, although several trials are under way to try to determine the most effective and safest manner to remove patients with type II diabetes from insulin. In general, if a patient is taking less than 40 to 50 units of insulin a day, then the success of achieving adequate control on oral agents alone is good. Additional clinical characteristics that may indicate success in taking patients off insulin include:

- Duration of diabetes less than 10 to 15 years
- Normal or above ideal body weight

- Glucose toxicity not present, ie, fasting blood glucose values < 200 mg/dL and/or postprandial blood glucose < 250 mg/dL
- Diabetes diagnosed after age 35.

It is important to emphasize that these characteristics are not written in stone and should be used only as guidelines.

If a patient is on a combination of a daytime oral antidiabetic agent and bedtime insulin, then adding either metformin, acarbose, or a sulfonylurea during the day may prove effective. When the new oral agent is started, the patient's insulin dose should be reduced by one third to one half, depending on the degree of glycemic control at the time of the attempted switchover. As the dose of the oral agent is increased, usually to the maximum dose, the insulin could be further reduced and eventually discontinued, depending on the home glucose readings.

In order to ensure safety, the patient should:
- Be reliable
- Be competent at home glucose monitoring
- Have ready telephone access to his/her caregiver.

REFERENCES

1. Reichard P, Nilsson BY, Rosenqvist U. The effect of long-term intensified insulin treatment on the development of microvascular complications of diabetes mellitus. *N Engl J Med*. 1993;329:304-309.

2. The Diabetes Control and Complications Trial Research Group. The effect of intensive treatment of diabetes on the development and progression of long-term complications in insulin-dependent diabetes mellitus. *N Engl J Med*. 1993;329:977-986.

3. American Diabetes Association. *Medical Management of Non–insulin-dependent (Type II) Diabetes*, 3rd ed. Alexandria, Va: American Diabetes Association; 1994:40-49.

4. DeFronzo RA, Goodman AM, The Multicenter Metformin Study Group. Efficacy of metformin in patients with non–insulin-dependent diabetes mellitus. *N Engl J Med*. 1995; 333:541-549.

5. Chiasson JL, Josse RG, Hunt JA, et al. The efficacy of acarbose in the treatment of patients with non–insulin-dependent diabetes mellitus. *Ann Intern Med*. 1994;121: 928-935.

6. Consensus Statement. The pharmacologic treatment of hyperglycemia in NIDDM. *Diabetes Care*. 1996;19:S54-S61.

7. Coniff RF, Shapiro JA, Seaton TB, Bray GA. Multicenter, placebo-controlled trial comparing acarbose (BAY g 5421) with placebo, tolbutamide and tolbutamide-plus-acarbose in non–insulin-dependent diabetes mellitus. *Am J Med*. 1995; 98:443-451.

8. Nolan JJ, Ludvik B, Beerdsen P, Joyce M, Olefsky J. Improvement in glucose tolerance and insulin resistance in obese subjects treated with troglitazone. *N Engl J Med*. 1994;331:1188-1193.

8 Insulin Therapy

Insulin therapy should be reserved for patients who have failed an adequate trial of diet, exercise, and oral antidiabetic agents. Many insulin regimens are recommended, although it is not clear from the literature which regimen is best. This chapter will focus on the different insulin regimens commonly used to normalize glucose levels and glycosylated hemoglobin in patients with type II diabetes mellitus.

Based on the natural history of type II diabetes, many people will eventually require therapy with insulin. The period of time before insulin is required tends to be highly variable and is based on numerous factors. The most important explanation is the extent of beta cell exhaustion resulting in relative endogenous insulinopenia. This leads to progressive loss of compensatory hyperinsulinemia, which is required to achieve and maintain a sufficient degree of glycemic control, especially in patients taking oral hypoglycemic agents. In other cases, obesity, pregnancy, or any number of medications, as well as a variety of medical illnesses, may exacerbate the insulin-resistant state and convert a patient previously well controlled on oral agents to one requiring insulin.

In addition to the natural history of type II diabetes, there is heterogeneity in its pathophysiology, which may influence when patients require insulin. Some patients diagnosed with type II diabetes may actually be closer to insulin-dependent or type I diabetes with severe insulinopenia. Many of these patients have been shown to have islet cell antibody (ICA) positivity or antibodies to glutamic acid decarboxylase (GAD), with a decreased C-peptide response to glucagon stimulation and a propensity for primary oral medication failure. There are also wide geographic and racial differences that may influence the need for insulin therapy. For example, Asian patients with type II diabetes tend to be thinner, to be diagnosed with diabetes at an earlier age, to fail oral hypoglycemic agents much sooner, and to be more sensitive to insulin therapy than the classic centrally obese patient in the United States.

Insulin therapy can improve or correct many of the metabolic abnormalities present in patients with type II diabetes mellitus. Exogenous insulin administration significantly reduces glucose levels by suppressing hepatic glucose production, increasing postprandial glucose utilization, and improving the abnormal lipoprotein levels and composition commonly seen in patients with insulin resistance. Insulin therapy may also decrease or eliminate the effects of glucose toxicity by reducing hyperglycemia to improve insulin sensitivity and beta cell secretory function.

Selecting an Insulin Preparation

A wide variety of purified insulins are available, including beef and pork, although human insulin is becoming the predominant form used. In addition, insulin lispro (Humalog), the fast-activity insulin analog, is now available for clinical use. Human insulin is particularly useful for patients with:
- Insulin allergy
- Severe insulin resistance caused by insulin antibodies
- Lipoatrophy
- A requirement for intermittent insulin therapy (ie, during pregnancy and acute problems such as infection, myocardial infarction, and emergency surgery).

Many of the complications of insulin therapy are now uncommon because of the advent of more purified preparations.

Selecting an appropriate insulin preparation also depends on the desired time course of action or pharmacokinetics. The values shown in Table 8.1 are general guidelines that can vary considerably among individuals, especially those with type II diabetes. Other factors that influence the action of insulin within an individual include:

- Site and depth of injection
- Skin temperature
- Exercise.

The recommended interval between insulin injection and mealtime is 30 minutes when the preprandial blood glucose is adequate (less than 140 mg/dL). The patient should wait longer if the blood glucose is higher. Proper timing of the premeal injection will markedly improve the postprandial blood glucose level and possibly reduce the incidence of delayed hypoglycemia. Eating within a few minutes of the injection, or before the injection, markedly reduces the ability of the insulin to prevent a rapid rise in blood glucose and may increase the risk of delayed hypoglycemia. Common insulin regimens used in adult diabetes are listed in Table 8.2.

Application of Intensive Insulin Therapy

The goals of therapy should be individually tailored. Candidates for intensive management should be:

- Motivated
- Compliant
- Educable

TABLE 8.1 — TIME COURSE OF ACTION OF INSULIN PREPARATIONS

Insulin Preparation	Onset of Action	Peak Action	Duration of Action
Short-acting (regular)	30 min	2-5 h	5-8 h
Insulin analogs (Humalog)	Minutes	45 min	4-5 h
Intermediate-acting (NPH or Lente)	1-3 h	6-12 h	16-24 h
Long-acting (Ultralente)	4-6 h	8-20 h	24-28 h
Mixtures (70/30, 50/50)	30 min	7-12 h	16-24 h

This table summarizes the typical time course of action of various insulin preparations. These values are highly variable among individuals. Even in a given patient, these values vary depending on the site and depth of injection, skin temperature, and exercise.

Abbreviations: NPH, neutral protamine Hagedorn.

Source: Adapted from American Diabetes Association. *Medical Management of Non–insulin-dependent (Type II) Diabetes*, 3rd ed. Alexandria, Va: American Diabetes Association; 1994:45.

TABLE 8.2 — COMMON INSULIN REGIMENS USED IN ADULT DIABETES

Regimen	Administration	Comment
Single insulin injections	NPH or Lente alone or with regular insulin at breakfast, supper, or bedtime depending on home glucose monitoring results	Increase dose every 3 to 5 days; glucose control usually inadequate with single injection therapy
Insulin and oral agents	NPH or Lente at bedtime or before supper added to maximal-dose oral antidiabetic agents	Total oral dose can be given before breakfast if predinner blood glucose values remain elevated
Multiple insulin injections	NPH or Lente with regular insulin prebreakfast and supper; regular insulin before meals and NPH, Lente or Ultralente at bedtime or late afternoon	Premixed 70/30 prebreakfast and predinner is useful, especially in obese patients

Abbreviation: NPH, neutral protamine Hagedorn.

Source: Reprinted with permission from Henry RR, Edelman SV. Metabolic disorders. Diabetes mellitus in adults. In: Rakel RE, ed. *Conn's Current Therapy*. Philadelphia: WB Saunders; 1996:526.

8

- Without other medical conditions and physical limitations that preclude accurate and reliable self-monitoring of capillary blood glucose (SMCBG) and insulin administration.

In addition, caution is advised in patients who are elderly or who are unaware of the signs of hypoglycemia. Other limitations to achieving normoglycemia may include high titers of insulin antibodies, especially in those patients with a prior history of intermittent insulin use of animal origin. The site of insulin injection may also change the pharmacokinetics, and absorption can be highly variable, especially if lipohypertrophy is present. The periumbilical area has been shown to be one of the most desirable areas to inject insulin because of the rapid and consistent absorption kinetics observed at this location.

Prior to initiating insulin therapy, the patient should be well educated in the:
- Techniques of SMCBG
- Proper insulin administration
- Self adjustment of insulin dose if appropriate
- Dietary and exercise strategies.

The patient and family members also need to be informed about hypoglycemia prevention, recognition, and treatment. Initial and ongoing education by a diabetes management team is crucial for long-term success and safety.

Combination Therapy

Combination therapy usually refers to the use of oral antidiabetic agents together with a single injection of intermediate-acting insulin at bedtime. The rationale for using an evening insulin strategy is based on the pathophysiology of fasting hyperglycemia in type II diabetes. The underlying tenet for combination therapy assumes that if evening insulin lowers the fasting glucose level to normal levels, then the daytime oral agent will be more effective at controlling postprandial hyperglycemia and maintaining euglycemia throughout the day. Metabolic profiles in type II diabetes have clearly demonstrated that the fasting blood glucose contributes more to daytime hyperglycemia than do postprandial changes. In addition, the fasting blood glucose level is highly correlated with the degree of hepatic glucose production during the early morning hours. Bedtime intermediate-acting insulin's peak action coincides with the onset of the dawn phenomenon (early morning resistance to insulin caused by diurnal variations in growth hormone and possibly norepinephrine levels), which usually occurs between 3:00 and 7:00 AM.

Patient selection is very important when considering combination therapy. The question of whether a patient is still responding in a satisfactory manner to oral antidiabetic agents such as sulfonylureas is of primary importance. Patients have a higher likelihood of success using daytime oral agents and bedtime insulin if they:

- Are obese
- Have had overt diabetes for less than 10 to 15 years
- Are diagnosed with type II diabetes after the age of 35
- Do not have fasting blood glucose values consistently over 250 to 300 mg/dL
- Have evidence of endogenous insulin secretory ability.

Although standard measurement conditions and levels for C-peptide have not been established for this clinical situation, a fasting (0.2 nmol/L) or glucagon-stimulated (> 0.40 nmol/L) C-peptide value indicates some degree of endogenous insulin secretory ability.

Patients with type II diabetes diagnosed under the age of 35 more often have atypical forms of diabetes. Subjects with diabetes longer than 10 to 15 years in duration tend to have a greater chance of beta cell exhaustion and thus be less responsive to the oral hypoglycemic agents.

Thin patients are more likely to be hypoinsulinemic and often respond inadequately to oral sulfonylureas, which leads to combination-therapy failure. In addition, when the fasting glucose level becomes markedly elevated, this is often associated with a concomitant decrease in endogenous insulin secretory ability, which renders oral agents ineffective. The actual number of patients who might fit into this category and possibly respond to combination therapy is unknown but is estimated to be between 20% and 30% of all patients "failing" maximum doses of oral agent therapy.

There are also a number of practical reasons why combination therapy may be beneficial (Table 8.2):

- The patient does not need to learn how to mix different types of insulin
- Hospitalization is not required
- Patient compliance and acceptance are better with single rather than multiple injections of insulin.

Combination therapy also requires a lower total dose of exogenous insulin than a full two- or three-injection-a-day regimen. This usually contributes to less weight gain and peripheral hyperinsulinemia.

Calculation of the initial bedtime intermediate-acting insulin dose can be based on clinical judgment or on various formulas using fasting blood glucose level or body weight. For example, one can divide the average fasting blood glucose (mg/dL) by 18 or divide the body weight in kilograms by 10 to calculate the initial dose of NPH or Lente insulin to be started at bedtime.[1] One can also safely start 5 to 10 units of intermediate-acting insulin for thin patients and 10 to 15 units for obese patients at bedtime as an initial estimated dose. In either case, the dose is increased in 2 to 5 unit increments every 3 to 4 days until the morning fasting blood glucose level is consistently in the range of 70 to 140 mg/dL (Table 8.3).

The most ideal time to give the evening injection of intermediate-acting insulin is between 10 PM and midnight. Many reliable patients can make their own adjustments using SMCBG. Table 8.4 demonstrates a patient self-instruction sheet for bedtime insulin adjustments. Once the fasting blood glucose levels are consistently in a desirable range, the prelunch, predinner, and bedtime blood glucose must be monitored to determine if the oral hypoglycemic agents are maintaining daytime euglycemia.

Based on the results of SMCBG, combination therapy can be altered to reduce hyperglycemia at identified times during the day. For example, a common situation seen with daytime sulfonylureas and bedtime intermediate-acting insulin is an improvement in the fasting, prelunch, and predinner blood glucose, although the postdinner blood glucose level remains excessively high (> 200 mg/dL). In this clinical situation, an injection of premixed regular and intermediate-acting insulin (ie, 70/30 insulin) predinner instead of the bedtime dose of intermediate-acting insulin may be more efficacious. This regimen will often improve the postdinner blood glucose values, because the premixed insulin contains rapidly acting regular insulin yet will still allow overnight glucose control secondary to the intermediate-acting component. With this regimen, however, one must be more cautious of early morning hypoglycemia because the intermediate insulin given before dinner will exert its peak effect earlier. This latter concern has not been a major clinical problem in patients with type II diabetes compared with those with type I diabetes mellitus.

TABLE 8.3 — GUIDELINES FOR DOSING INSULIN IN COMBINATION THERAPY

1. To calculate insulin dose (NPH or Lente): divide average fasting blood glucose (mg/dL) by 18 or divide body weight (kg) by 10 to calculate initial dose of NPH or Lente insulin for bedtime (10:00 PM to midnight).

2. Initial bedtime dose for lean patients: 5-10 U intermediate-acting insulin.

3. Initial bedtime dose for obese patients: 10-15 U intermediate-acting insulin.

4. Increase dose of insulin in increments of 2-5 U every 3-4 days until the AM fasting blood glucose level is consistently 70-140 mg/dL (reliable patients can make their own adjustments using results from home glucose monitoring).

5. Patients continue taking the maximum dose of their oral agents; if daytime glucose levels become too low (< 100 mg/dL), the dose of the oral agent must be decreased.

6. If the oral agent cannot maintain daytime euglycemia, the oral agent must be stopped and conventional insulin therapy must be started.

Abbreviation: NPH, neural protamine Hagedorn.

It is recommended that after addition of evening insulin, patients remain on their maximal dose of oral antidiabetic agent. If the daytime blood glucose levels start to become excessively low, the dose of oral medication must be adjusted downward. This is not an uncommon scenario because glucose toxicity may be reduced as a result of improved glucose control, leading to enhanced sensitivity to both oral agents and insulin. If the prelunch and predinner blood glucose levels remain excessively high on combination therapy, the oral antidiabetic agent is likely not contributing significantly to glycemic control throughout the day.

TABLE 8.4 — PATIENT SELF ADJUSTMENT OF EVENING INSULIN

1. Begin with a dose of _____ units of NPH insulin administered just before bedtime.

2. If the prebreakfast blood sugar is > 140 mg/dL for 3 days in a row, then increase the evening NPH insulin dose by _____ units.

3. If the prebreakfast blood sugar is < 80 mg/dL for 2 days in a row, then decrease the evening NPH insulin by _____ units.

4. Remember not to increase the insulin dose more frequently than every 3 days.

5. If you have any questions, please call me at _____.

6. Provider's name:_____.

_____
Physician/Nurse Practitioner

In this situation, a more conventional two-injection-a-day regimen should be employed while discontinuing the oral antidiabetic agents.

In summary, combination therapy can be a simple and effective tool to normalize glycemia and glycosylated hemoglobin levels in selected patients with type II diabetes mellitus failing oral antidiabetic agents. The most common clinical situation where combination therapy can be successful is in the patient failing sulfonylurea therapy but with some evidence of responsiveness to the oral agents. Bedtime intermediate-acting insulin is given and progressively increased so as to normalize the fasting blood glucose level. When the fasting blood glucose level is brought under control, the success of combination therapy is dependent on the ability of the daytime oral antidiabetic agents to maintain euglycemia. If this cannot be achieved, then the oral hypoglycemic agents should be stopped and conventional insulin regimens employed.

Multiple Injection Regimens

One of the most common insulin regimens utilized in type II diabetes mellitus is a split-mixed regimen consisting of a prebreakfast and predinner dose of an intermediate- and fast-acting insulin. This split-mixed two-injection-a-day regimen is often inadequate for patients with type I diabetes mellitus and results in persistent early morning hypoglycemia and fasting hyperglycemia. Such problems do not appear to occur as frequently in type II diabetes. This is likely because of pathophysiologic differences between type I and type II diabetes, particularly in:
- Endogenous insulin secretory ability
- Insulin resistance
- Counterregulatory mechanisms.

There are a number of important aspects about intensive glucose control with insulin in obese patients with type II diabetes:
- First, the average daily dose of insulin needed to control such patients may approximate one unit per kilogram of body weight.
- Second, the total daily insulin requirement can successfully be split equally between the prebreakfast and predinner injections.
- Third, obese patients will require approximately 70% of their total insulin requirement as NPH or Lente with the remainder as regular insulin.
- Fourth, the split-mixed regimen in patients with type II diabetes is usually devoid of the common problems seen with this regimen in type I diabetes, particularly early morning hypoglycemia and fasting (preprandial) hyperglycemia.
- Fifth, mild and severe hypoglycemic events are much less frequent in patients with type II diabetes mellitus compared with patients with

type I diabetes undergoing intensive insulin therapy.

- Finally, weight gain with peripheral hyper-insulinemia frequently occurs in type II diabetes and may contribute to metabolic and vascular complications.

In most cases, single-injection therapy with an intermediate- or long-acting insulin has been shown to be inadequate to normalize glycosylated hemoglobin and maintain 24-hour euglycemia in type II diabetes.

There are several acceptable methods to initiate insulin therapy in type II diabetes. A conservative yet effective strategy utilizing a step-wise approach to instituting a split-mixed regimen is given in Table 8.5. A simple alternative method to initiating a split-mixed regimen in obese patients uses 70/30 premixed insulin with an initial total daily insulin dose (0.4-0.8 units/kg) equally split between the prebreakfast and predinner injections. Adjustments are made based on SMCBG results, which may dictate the need to change the ratio of intermediate- to regular-acting insulin either upward or downward. For morbidly obese patients, the insulin requirements rise almost exponentially as ideal body weight increases above 150%. In contrast, caution should be used when starting thin patients with type II diabetes on insulin, especially premixed insulins with fixed doses of regular insulin (total daily dose 0.2-0.5 units/kg). This group tends to be more sensitive to the glucose-lowering effects and thus more prone to severe hypoglycemia. If a multiple insulin injection regimen or subcutaneous insulin pump therapy is to be initiated, Ultralente should be used to provide a steady basal rate of insulin bioavailability. This component should constitute approximately 50% to 60% of the total daily insulin requirements. Premeal boluses of regular insulin are also given with adjustment based on the 2-hour postprandial blood glucose measurements.

8

TABLE 8.5 — STEPWISE APPROACH FOR INITIATING A SPLIT-MIXED INSULIN REGIMEN IN PATIENTS WITH TYPE II DIABETES

1. **First Goal: fasting BG 80 mg/dL to 120 mg/dL**
   Initial dose of NPH insulin: 0.2 U/kg before dinner.
   Change dose of evening NPH insulin based on subsequent fasting BG as follows:
   - If BG > 180 mg/dL, increase by 0.5 U/kg
   - If BG 120 mg/dL to 180 md/dL, increase by 0.05 U/kg
   - If BG 80 mg/dL to 120 mg/dL, no change in dose
   - If BG < 80 mg/dL, decrease by 0.1 U/kg.

2. **Second Goal: predinner BG 80 mg/dL to 120 mg/dL**
   Initial dose of NPH insulin before breakfast and criteria for adjustment same as for first goal, except based on subsequent predinner BG.
   Proceed to third goal only after first and second goals are achieved.

3. **Third Goal: postprandial (2-h) BG < 180 md/dL (after breakfast and dinner)**
   Change each dose of regular insulin based on subsequent postprandial (2-h) BG as follows:
   - If BG > 180 mg/dL, increase by 0.025 U/kg
   - If BG 120 mg/dL to 180 mg/dL, no change in dose
   - If BG 80 mg/dL to 120 mg/dL, decrease by 0.025 U/kg
   - If BG < 80 mg/dL increase dose by 0.05 U/kg

   All injections should be given subcutaneously in the periumbilical region 30 minutes before breakfast and dinner.

Abbreviation: BG, blood glucose; U, units.

Source: Adapted from Henry RR, Edelman SV. Metabolic disorders. Diabetes mellitus in adults. In: Rakel RE, ed. *Conn's Current Therapy*. Philadelphia: WB Saunders Co; 1996:526.

In summary, there is no one perfect insulin regimen that can be used in type II diabetes. In a subgroup of patients failing maximum doses of sulfonylureas, combination therapy can:

- Be beneficial
- Be easy to administer
- Reduce the need for large doses of exogenous insulin.

Once a patient demonstrates unresponsiveness to combination therapy, however, a more conventional insulin regimen should be employed. When failure to combination therapy occurs, a split-mixed regimen of intermediate- and regular-acting insulin given prebreakfast and predinner is usually preferred. Insulin adjustments are based on SMCBG and premixed insulins are easy to administer and effective.

Particular attention should be directed toward minimizing the weight gain seen with intensive insulin therapy. Obese patients failing combination therapy usually require large amounts of insulin and are susceptible to weight gain, which may make therapeutic success more difficult. Normalizing glycosylated hemoglobin with a particular regimen is dependent on numerous variables including:

- The severity of insulin resistance
- The extent and type of obesity
- Prior failure on oral hypoglycemic agents
- Preceding degree of glucose control
- Other complicating medical conditions.

Furthermore, the success of a particular insulin regimen is influenced by the severity of glucose toxicity. Prolonged hyperglycemia reduces beta cell secretory ability and worsens peripheral insulin resistance. Thus, the metabolic success of these different insulin regimens can be highly variable.

External Subcutaneous Insulin Infusion Pumps

Continuous subcutaneous insulin infusion (CSII) has been used primarily in patients with type I diabetes. Although there are few clinical trials using CSII in patients with type II diabetes, beneficial metabolic effects have been demonstrated in this population. An external insulin pump can be useful for patients who have been unable to achieve euglycemia with three or four daily injections of insulin or whose lifestyle requires greater flexibility in terms of meal schedules and daily activities, including travel. CSII is most appropriate in thin, insulin-requiring type II diabetics unable to reach adequate glycemic control with a multiple injection regimen.

Candidates for CSII must be highly motivated to improve their glucose control. They need to be willing to work closely with their health-care providers and assume substantial responsibility for their daily care. These patients must also be capable of understanding and demonstrating accurate use of an insulin pump as well as SMCBG in order to make appropriate insulin adjustments.

Insulin Analogs

DNA technology has allowed the development of insulin analogs that more closely mimic the physiologic meal-related action of insulin.[2] Insulin lispro (Humalog) is now available for clinical use in the United States. Subcutaneous administration of insulin analogs immediately before a meal provides a more rapid and predictable onset of action and clearance.

Insulin lispro is rapidly absorbed at the injection site. The onset of action is nearly immediate, peaking

in action about 45 minutes after injection, with rapid disappearance from the circulation. Benefits include:
- Improved postprandial glucose control
- Greater lifestyle flexibility in terms of premeal injection timing (recommended to be taken 5 minutes before a meal)
- Reductions in episodes of delayed hypoglycemia.

Insulin lispro may also have particular advantages in the obese, insulin-requiring type II diabetic because of its greater potency, more rapid onset of action, and faster clearance.

Complications of Insulin Therapy

Weight gain and hypoglycemia are the most frequently reported complications of insulin therapy. Both can be minimized with appropriate preventive measures and dosage adjustments.

■ Weight Gain

Hyperinsulinemia caused by large amounts of exogenous insulin can lead to marked increases in weight, which is a real concern in type II diabetes. Obesity itself is an insulin-resistant state that contributes to a cycle of worsening insulin resistance, increasing insulin requirements, and further weight gain. Some patients, particularly the obese, may require large doses of insulin to normalize glycemia in order to overcome the insulin resistance that is typical of type II diabetes. The additional exogenous insulin can result in hyperinsulinemia and an average increase in body weight of 3% to 9%. Excessive weight gain can be minimized by using the lowest possible dose of insulin to achieve target glycemic goals and encouraging the patient to decrease caloric intake and increase exercise.

Another consideration is the theoretical relationship between prolonged circulating hyperinsulinemia and the corresponding potential for accelerated development of atherosclerosis. Although a direct cause-effect relationship has not been established, the strong association between these two conditions should not be ignored.

■ Hypoglycemia

The incidence of hypoglycemic reaction increases with insulin therapy, particularly intensive regimens, and the thin and the elderly are most affected by such episodes. Obese patients with type II diabetes tend to have much less hypoglycemia than those with type I diabetes. Severe hypoglycemia is rare in obese patients with type II diabetes and is usually related to causal factors such as:

- Overinsulinization
- Underfeeding
- Unplanned strenuous physical activity
- Excessive alcohol.

Frequent SMCBG by the patient with adjustment in the dose or type of insulin can significantly reduce the likelihood of hypoglycemia.

REFERENCES

1. Edelman SV, Henry RR. Insulin therapy for normalizing the glycosylated hemoglobin in type II diabetes: applications, benefits and risks. *Diabetes Review*. 1994;3:308-334.

2. Upcoming diabetes medications. In: *Diabetes Monitor*. Independence, Mo: Midwest Diabetes Care Center; April, 1996.

9   Treatment Algorithm

The primary treatment goals of managing type II diabetes are to:
- Eliminate symptoms of hyperglycemia
- Achieve and maintain normal or near-normal metabolic and biochemical parameters (both fasting and postprandial blood glucose levels, glycated hemoglobin [Table 9.1], fasting low-density lipoprotein [LDL] and high-density lipoprotein [HDL] cholesterol, and triglycerides)
- Assist the patient in achieving and maintaining a reasonable body weight
- Prevent or delay the development and progression of microvascular and macrovascular complications.

Therapeutic efforts to achieve these goals involve using a variety of treatment modalities:
- Dietary modifications
- Regular physical activity
- Oral antidiabetic agents
- Insulin injections.

An individualized approach is recommended based on:
- Patient age
- The presence of coexisting illnesses and/or diabetes-related complications
- Lifestyle, including:
  - Attitudes
  - Habits
  - Cultural/ethnic status
- Financial considerations
- Ability to learn and follow self-management skills
- Level of patient motivation.

TABLE 9.1 — RECOMMENDED LEVELS OF GLUCOSE CONTROL

Biochemical Parameters	Normal (nondiabetic)	Acceptable	Action Recommended
Fasting/preprandial glucose	< 115 mg/dL	80-120 mg/dL	< 80 mg/dL or > 140 mg/dL
Bedtime glucose	< 120 mg/dL	100-140 mg/dL	< 100 mg/dL or > 160 mg/dL
Postprandial glucose	< 140	140-180 mg/dL	>180 mg/dL
Glycated hemoglobin*	< 6%	< 7%	> 8%

* Hemoglobin A_{1C} is referenced to a nondiabetic range of 4% to 6% (mean 5%, SD 0.5%).

Adapted from: American Diabetes Association. *Medical Management of Non–insulin-dependent (Type II) Diabetes*, 3rd ed. Alexandria, Va: American Diabetes Association; 1994:26.

The cornerstone of effective diabetes management is maintaining good glycemic control. Compelling evidence indicates that long-term glycemic control can prevent or delay the microvascular complications of diabetes. The Diabetes Control and Complications Trial (DCCT)[3] demonstrated definitively the value of intensive therapy of patients with type I diabetes in delaying the onset and slowing the progression of retinopathy, nephropathy, and neuropathy. Although this large, multicenter study did not include patients with type II diabetes, hyperglycemia is likely to be associated with the development and progression of microvascular complications in type II diabetes as well as in type I diabetes.[4] Therefore, the benefits of reducing glycemia can be reasonably extrapolated to patients with type II diabetes.

Currently, results are pending from randomized clinical trials, similar to the DCCT, evaluating the merit of near-normalization of blood glucose in type II diabetes. However, despite the absence of confirmatory data, the American Diabetes Association (ADA) has indicated that patients with type II diabetes are likely to benefit from similar improvements in glycemic control. The ADA now recommends establishing a management goal of achieving the best possible blood glucose control in patients with type II diabetes.[4] Treatment methods for managing type II diabetes should focus on:

- Dietary modifications
- Exercise
- Weight control
- Supplemental oral hypoglycemic agents and/or insulin as needed.

The following algorithm (Figure 9.1) provides a general guideline for making decisions regarding the various types of pharmacologic therapy.

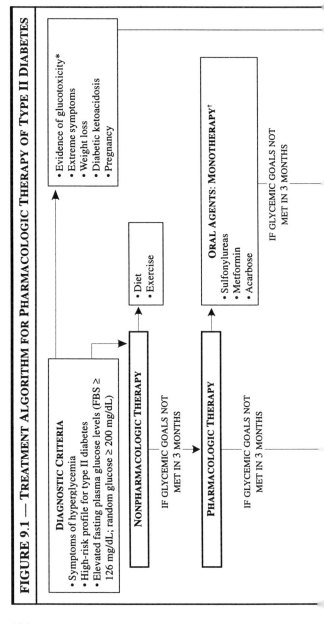

FIGURE 9.1 — TREATMENT ALGORITHM FOR PHARMACOLOGIC THERAPY OF TYPE II DIABETES

DIAGNOSTIC CRITERIA
- Symptoms of hyperglycemia
- High-risk profile for type II diabetes
- Elevated fasting plasma glucose levels (FBS ≥ 126 mg/dL; random glucose ≥ 200 mg/dL)

- Evidence of glucotoxicity*
- Extreme symptoms
- Weight loss
- Diabetic ketoacidosis
- Pregnancy

NONPHARMACOLOGIC THERAPY
- Diet
- Exercise

IF GLYCEMIC GOALS NOT MET IN 3 MONTHS

PHARMACOLOGIC THERAPY

IF GLYCEMIC GOALS NOT MET IN 3 MONTHS

ORAL AGENTS: MONOTHERAPY†
- Sulfonylureas
- Metformin
- Acarbose

IF GLYCEMIC GOALS NOT MET IN 3 MONTHS

ORAL AGENTS: COMBINED THERAPY[†]

- Sulfonylurea + metformin
- Sulfonylurea + acarbose
- Metformin + acarbose
- Sulfonylurea + metformin + acarbose

COMBINED: INSULIN + ORAL AGENT[†]

- Single bedtime intermediate-acting insulin (adjusted to reduce FBS to < 140 mg/dL consistently) plus daytime oral agent

IF DAYTIME GLYCEMIA NOT ACHIEVED IN 3 MONTHS, DISCONTINUE ORAL AGENT

INSULIN THERAPY

INSULIN ALONE[‡]

- Split-mixed regimen: intermediate- and fast-acting (70/30), prebreakfast and predinner
- Multiple injections (3 or more)
- Continuous subcutaneous insulin infusion (CSII)

---

* Insulin use may be temporary to reduce glucotoxicity; patient then may respond to sulfonylureas and other oral agents.
† Choice of therapy depends on individual patient characteristics.
‡ Choice of insulin regimen based on individual assessment.

9

REFERENCES

1. American Diabetes Association. *Medical Management of Non–insulin-dependent (Type II) Diabetes*, 3rd ed. Alexandria, Va: American Diabetes Association; 1994:22-39.

2. American Diabetes Association. Position statement. Standards of medical care for patients with diabetes mellitus. *Diabetes Care*. 1991;14:10-13.

3. American Diabetes Association. Clinical practice recommendations 1995. Standards of medical care for patients with diabetes mellitus. *Diabetes Care*. 1995;18(suppl 1):8-15.

4. Ohkubo Y, Kishikawa H, Araki E, et al. Intensive insulin therapy prevents the progression of diabetic microvascular complications in Japanese patients with non–insulin-dependent diabetes mellitus: a randomized prospective 6-year study. *Diabetes Res Clin Pract*. 1995;28:103-117.

10 Assessment of the Treatment Regimen

Certain key clinical and metabolic parameters should be monitored during office visits:[1]
- To assess glycemic control:
  - Glycosylated hemoglobin level
  - Plasma glucose values
- To assess cardiovascular risk:
  - Lipoprotein analysis
  - Blood pressure
  - Body weight
- To assess for evidence of diabetic complications.

The metabolic goals for these parameters are shown in Table 10.1.[2]

Glycemic control is assessed during office visits with determinations of plasma glucose levels and assays for glycated hemoglobin. Patients can evaluate the effects of their treatment regimen on a day-to-day basis between office visits by using self-monitoring of capillary blood glucose (SMCBG) at home. A combination of physician and patient assessment methods is used to obtain the most accurate information about the degree of metabolic control.

Measuring Plasma Glucose Concentrations

Day-to-day glycemic control is reflected in measurements of plasma glucose concentrations. However, because this measurement is an isolated finding at a single point in time, it may not represent a patient's

TABLE 10.1 — METABOLIC GOALS OF EFFECTIVE MANAGEMENT

- Glycosylated hemoglobin
  - Within 1 percentage point above the upper range of normal
  - Within 3 SD from the mean
- Fasting plasma glucose level between 70 mg/dL and 120 mg/dL
- Two-hour postprandial plasma glucose level < 180 mg/dL
- Systolic/diastolic blood pressure < 130/85 mmHg
- Approach or maintain ideal body weight
- Lipoprotein goals
  - Triglyceride level < 200 mg/dL
  - HDL cholesterol level > 35 mg/dL
  - LDL cholesterol level < 100 mg/dL
  - Total cholesterol level < 200 mg/dL, although this level may be misleading in patients with type II diabetes

Goals for blood pressure are different if the patient has evidence of ischemic heart disease. Lipoprotein goals follow current National Cholesterol Education Program Guidelines.

Source: Edelman SV, Henry RR. Insulin therapy for normalizing glycosylated hemoglobin in type II diabetes: application, benefits, and risks. *Diabetes Reviews*. 1994;3:310.

usual metabolic state. Some limitations of plasma glucose measurements are:[1]

- It is difficult to know the meaning of a single random or fasting plasma glucose determination.
- Random determinations may reflect peak, trough, or values in-between because of the wide daily variations in glucose levels.
- The stress of an office visit may result in higher-than-usual glucose values.

- Some patients may become atypically adherent to their treatment regimen or use extra insulin before an office visit, resulting in an uncharacteristically low glucose level.
- The presence of an intercurrent illness at the time of an office visit (which often is the case) can alter blood glucose levels.

Home glucose monitoring data are appropriate for assessing glycemic control and making changes in the therapeutic regimen of patients being treated with diet, oral agents, and insulin therapy. Inaccurate or suspicious results would be revealed by a glycated hemoglobin assay, which reflects the level of glucose control for the preceding 2 to 3 months. Because a single plasma glucose measurement does not provide an adequate assessment of any type of therapy, other corroborating data are needed such as symptoms of hypoglycemia or uncontrolled diabetes, a glycated hemoglobin value, and repeated plasma glucose measurements.

The timing of plasma glucose measurements has an impact on the significance of the findings:[2]

- A postprandial sample obtained 1 to 2 hours after a patient has eaten is the most sensitive measurement because glucose levels are the highest during this time; total carbohydrate content of the meal will be reflected in this glucose value.
- A postprandial or fasting plasma glucose level reflects how efficiently carbohydrates from a meal have been cleared from the plasma.

Measuring Glycated Hemoglobin

Assays of $HgbA_1$, $HgbA_{1c}$, and glycated hemoglobin are used extensively to provide an accurate time-integrated measure of average glycemic control over the previous 2 to 3 months and to correlate plasma glucose measurements and patients' SMCBG results. Because these assays do not reflect the glucose level at the time a blood sample is tested, measurements of glycated hemoglobin are not useful for making day-to-day adjustments in the treatment regimen.

Glycation refers to a carbohydrate-protein linkage. This irreversible process occurs as glucose in the plasma attaches itself to the hemoglobin component of red blood cells. Because the lifespan of red blood cells is 120 days, glycated hemoglobin assays reflect average blood glucose concentration over that time.

The amount of circulating glucose concentration to which the red cell is exposed influences the amount of glycated hemoglobin. Therefore, the hyperglycemia of diabetes causes an increase in the percentage of glycated hemoglobin in patients with diabetes; $HbgA_{1c}$ shows the greatest change, whereas the remaining glycated hemoglobins are relatively stable.

Levels of $HbgA_{1c}$ and $HgbA_{1}$ correlate best with the degree of diabetic control obtained several months earlier. Regardless of which assay is used, however, certain conditions can interfere with obtaining accurate results:[1]

- False low concentrations are likely in the presence of conditions that decrease the life of the red blood cell, such as:
  - Hemolytic anemia
  - Bleeding
  - Sickle cell trait.
- False high concentrations are likely in the presence of conditions that increase the lifespan of the red blood cell, eg, patients without a spleen. Other conditions that produce falsely elevated glycated hemoglobins include:
  - Uremia
  - High concentrations of fetal hemoglobin
  - High aspirin doses (> 10 g/day)
  - High concentrations of ethanol.

Regular monitoring of glycated hemoglobin (eg, every 3 to 6 months) is essential for all patients with diabetes regardless of their type of therapy. On a daily basis, patients typically measure capillary blood glucose levels before meals, postprandially, and at bedtime, particularly with intensive insulin regimens in which near-normal glycemia is being actively pursued. Even when preprandial levels seem satisfactory, patients' glycated hemoglobin results often are higher than expected. This finding would not have been evident through glucose measurements alone, and the need for further efforts to control blood glucose would not have been apparent without obtaining a glycated hemoglobin measurement.

Measuring Other Glycated Proteins

Enhanced glycation of other proteins occurs in diabetes and has been proposed as another method of assessing average glucose control. Because of the shorter half-life of serum proteins (17-20 days) compared with hemoglobin (56 days), measurement of serum fructosamine and affinity measurement of glycated albumin reflect a shorter period of average glucose control (2-3 weeks); both measurements are particularly useful for following patients with gestational diabetes. These tests might be expected to reveal changes in glucose control more quickly than a glycated hemoglobin assay. However, glycated albumin and glycated hemoglobin have been found to provide the equivalent results in insulin-requiring type II patients who have been stabilized. Consequently, tests of other glycated proteins reflect too brief a time period to be useful for most patients. Although the reliability and clinical applicability of these tests continue to be evaluated, measurement of glycated hemoglobin remains the preferred method.

Self-Monitoring of Capillary Blood Glucose (SMCBG)

This method of self-evaluation using capillary blood samples has become one of the most important tools for monitoring and improving glycemic control and making adjustments in the diabetes therapeutic regimen. SMCBG is a relatively painless procedure that involves pricking the finger with a lancet to obtain a drop of blood that is placed on a test strip. Reagents on the test strip contain an enzyme that causes glucose to react with a dye to produce a color change. The color intensity is proportional to the amount of glucose present. The test strip is placed in a small, hand-held meter that quantifies the glucose concentration using reflectance spectrometry. Some test strips can be read visually; other systems measure the electrical current produced by the glucose oxidation reaction to quantify the glucose concentration. Results obtained by SMCBG tend to have good agreement with plasma glucose concentrations obtained by clinical laboratory procedures if it is done properly. Patient technique tends to be the source of most discrepancies. Typically, plasma venous glucose measurements are within 15% of the results of whole blood capillary glucose determinations.

SMCBG is not a goal in itself but rather a means of achieving the goal of normal or near-normal glycemic control. It should be considered an important part of a comprehensive treatment regimen that includes:
- Diabetes education
- Counseling
- Management by a multidisciplinary team of health-care providers.

Goals of treatment and thus the reason for performing SMCBG must be clearly defined for the patient.

Patients must be motivated and capable of learning the proper techniques of SMCBG and committed to applying the results to modify their treatment. Healthcare providers must be able to discuss SMCBG results in a nonderogatory, helpful way that provides encouragement through open, honest communication and an atmosphere of support.

Reasons for Performing SMCBG

The following reasons for performing SMCBG have been outlined in a consensus statement by the American Diabetes Association:[3]

1. *To achieve or maintain a specific level of glycemic control* — As evidenced by results of the Diabetes Control and Complications Trial (DCCT),[4] intensive therapy that is closely monitored using SMCBG can help patients achieve near-normoglycemia and delay the onset and slow the progression of diabetic complications in type I diabetes, and likely in type II diabetes. Therefore, SMCBG at least 4 times daily is essential for evaluating and adjusting insulin doses in patients on intensive insulin regimens and, with lesser frequency, for patients on less complex insulin or combination regimens or those using oral agents and diet, directed toward achieving near-normoglycemia.

2. *To prevent and detect hypoglycemia* — Hypoglycemia is a major complication of treatment regimens, particularly those involving intensive application of pharmacologic therapy to achieve near-normoglycemia. The elderly are particularly susceptible to hypoglycemia, and certain oral antidiabetic agents such as the sulfonylureas can produce hypoglycemia. Therefore, appropriately timed SMCBG is the only way to detect asymptomatic hypoglycemia so that appropriate action

10

(adjusting insulin/oral agents, modifying diet/exercise) can be taken to prevent it from becoming severe.

3. *To avoid severe hyperglycemia* — Illness and certain drugs that alter insulin secretion (eg, phenytoin, thiazide diuretics) or insulin action (eg, prednisone) can increase the risk of severe hyperglycemia and/or ketoacidosis. SMCBG should be initiated or used more frequently in all of these situations to detect hyperglycemia before it becomes severe. In addition, patients on insulin therapy can use SMCBG data to adjust their insulin doses to avoid severe hyperglycemia.

4. *To adjust care in response to lifestyle changes in patients on pharmacologic therapy* — Glucose levels change in response to variations in diet and exercise. SMCBG can help identify patterns of response to planned exercise and daily activity and help modify pharmacologic therapy during times of increased or decreased caloric consumption.

Advantages and Disadvantages of SMCBG

SMCBG enables the patient to be involved in self-management and provides immediate feedback regarding the impact of diet, exercise, and pharmacologic therapy on blood glucose levels. Patients who are educated about SMCBG, how to use the results, and how to make self adjustments of insulin doses using algorithms (for insulin-requiring type II patients and type I patients) can achieve better daily glycemic control and have a better sense of self-control and participation in their own care. SMCBG also provides worthwhile feedback that the physician and other members of the diabetes health-care team can incorporate into ongoing evaluation of the treatment regimen. However, health-care professionals need to make a point of requesting and reviewing a patient's SMCBG data to provide helpful guidance and encouragement.

Advantages of SMCBG include:[5]

- Accurate, immediate results for detecting hypoglycemia and hyperglycemia
- Day-to-day assessment of glycemic control
- Follow-up information after changes in treatment to enhance accurate adjustments in pharmacologic therapy
- Enhanced patient independence, self-confidence, and participation in their treatment.

Disadvantages of SMCBG include:[5]

- Discomfort of lancing the finger to obtain blood
- Complexity of some testing procedures, requiring mental acuity and dexterity
- Potential malfunction of equipment that could lead to inaccurate results that may affect treatment decisions
- False results because of inaccurate technique that may affect treatment decisions.

SMCBG Systems

A combination of factors affect the overall performance of SMCBG systems:

- The analytic performance of the meter
- The ability of the user
- The quality of the test strips.

Analytic error can range from 4% to 33%; a goal of future SMCBG systems is an analytic error of ± 5%.[3] User performance is most affected by the quality and extent of training, which currently is hindered by reimbursement policies for diabetes education. Initial and regular assessments of a patient's SMCBG technique is necessary to assure accurate results. Patients need to be advised that test strips can be adversely affected by environmental factors. In addition, cautious use of generic test strips is warranted because of the complex process of calibrating test strips to specific meters.

Examples and features of available blood glucose meters are shown in Tables 10.2 and 10.3. The American Diabetes Association (ADA) Consensus Panel[3] advises periodic comparisons between a patient's SMCBG system and a sample obtained simultaneously and measured by a referenced laboratory .

Who Should Perform SMCBG?

Virtually all patients with diabetes should perform SMCBG because of the value of this evaluation tool in promoting improved glycemic control and reinforcing adherence to therapy. The frequency of SMCBG is dictated by the complexity of the therapeutic regimen. For example, insulin-using type II patients (particularly those on an intensive regimen) would need to perform more daily SMCBG evaluations than patients who are achieving acceptable glycemic control on diet, exercise, and oral agents.

Recommended Frequency of SMCBG

The frequency of SMCBG varies considerably based on the complexity of the therapeutic regimen and the clinical situation of the individual. In addition to guiding therapy, SMCBG also has educational and motivational advantages. For example, intermittent measurements 1 to 2 hours after meals can provide an assessment of glycemic response to various types of foods, thus helping patients learn which foods have the greatest and least impact on blood glucose, as well as how the size of a meal affects glucose levels. SMCBG also can help motivate patients (especially

116

obese patients trying to lose weight), because they can observe immediate decreases in their blood glucose levels in response to dietary modifications, exercise, and oral therapy.

Patients who demonstrate consistent, acceptable glucose results may require fewer tests (ie, one to three tests per week). However, testing requirements may increase when metabolic control worsens.

SMCBG for Patients Who Do Not Take Insulin

Traditionally, SMCBG was viewed as not necessary for type II patients on diet therapy or oral agents because glucose levels remained relatively stable on these treatment regimens. For these patients, SMCBG was recommended only for monitoring short-term adjustments in therapy or for patients at risk of hypoglycemia. Because better glycemic control has been shown to be associated with a greater frequency of SMCBG, this evaluation measure now is recommended for all patients, including those not taking insulin. The frequency of testing depends on how stable the patient is. Patients with less than optimal control should monitor their levels more frequently.

SMCBG recommendations for patients on diet therapy:
- Prebreakfast — two to three tests per week
- 2 hours postdinner — two to three tests per week.

Glucose values from these two important time points, in addition to a glycosylated hemoglobin value every 3 to 6 months, is an efficient way to follow patients on diet and oral agents.

SMCBG recommendations for patients using oral agents alone or combination therapy (daytime oral agents, evening insulin):

TABLE 10.2 — MEASURING THE METERS: SPECIFICATIONS

Product	Dimensions/ Weight	Strip Name/ Price (50 strips)	Wipe/ Nonwipe	Warranty	Calibration/Meter Performance Check	Power Source	Memory
Accu-Chek Advantage Boehringer-Mannheim Corp. (800) 858-8072	3.6" × 0.6" × 2.3" 3.0 oz	Advantage test strips $32-$35	Nonwipe; automatic timing	3 years	Advantage Code Key packaged with each new vial of strips.	Two 3-volt lithium coin-cell batteries	Stores 100 test results with date and time
Accu-Chek Easy Boehringer-Mannheim Corp. (800) 858-8072	4.5" × 2.5" × 0.8" 3.4 oz	Easy test strips $32-$35	Nonwipe; automatic timing	3 years	Easy Key Code Chip packaged with each new vial of strips; easy Check Kit provides electronic check	6-volt alkaline battery	Stores 350 test results with date and time
Accu-Chek Instant Boehringer-Mannheim Corp. (800) 858-8072	4.0" × 2.2" × 0.6" 1.8 oz	Accu-Chek Instant test strips $32-$35	Nonwipe; automatic timing	3 years	Push-bottom calibration	Four 1.5-volt alkaline batteries	Stores 9 test results
Accu-Chek III Boehringer-Mannheim Corp. (800) 858-8072	5.2" × 2.7" × 0.8" 4.8 oz	Chemstrip B for use with the Accu-Chek III $33-$36	Wipe; manual timing	2 years	Lot-specific code for each new vial; one-step calibration	6-volt alkaline battery	Stores 20 test results with date and time
Checkmate Plus Cascade Medical, Inc. (800) 525-6718	6.4" × 1.2" × 0.8" 2.1 oz	CheckMate Plus test strips $16	Nonwipe; automatic timing	Lifetime	Automatic; no codes or chips	Two 3-volt lithium batteries	Stores 255 test results with date and time

Diascan Partner Home Diagnostics, Inc. (800) 342-7226	8.4" × 3.1" × 0.6" 7.8 oz	Diascan test strips $30-$32	Wipe; manual timing	2 years	Lot-specific code for each new vial; push button to select code; check strip for daily meter performance check	6-volt J-cell battery	Stores 10 test results
Diascan-S Home Diagnostics, Inc. (800) 342-7226	5.2" × 3.1" × 0.6" 4.8 oz	Diascan test strips $30-$32	Wipe; manual timing	2 years	Lot-specific code for each new vial; push button to select code; check strip for daily meter performance check	6-volt J-cell battery	Stores 10 test results
Exactech Card Sensor MediSense, Inc. (800) 527-3339	3.7" × 2.2" × 0.4" 1.5 oz	ExacTech test strips $32-$35	Nonwipe; automatic timing	4 years	Calibration strip packaged in each box of strips	Nonreplaceable lithium batteries	Stores previous test result
Glucometer Elite Bayer Corp. Diagnostics Division (800) 348-8100	3.1" × 2.0" × 0.5" 1.8 oz	Glucometer Elite test strips $34	Nonwipe; automatic timing	5 years	Code strip with each new box of strips; check strip to confirm meter performance	Two 3-volt batteries	Stores 10 test results
Glucometer Encore Bayer Corp. Diagnostics Division (800) 348-8100	2.5" × 4.5" × 0.8" 3.6 oz	Glucometer Encore test strips $33-$34	Nonwipe; automatic timing	3 years	Lot-specific program number for each box of strips; push button to select program number; check "paddle" to confirm meter accuracy	Nonreplaceable battery	Stores 10 test results and average of stored test results

continued on next page →

10

Product	Dimensions/ Weight	Strip Name/ Price (50 strips)	Wipe/ Nonwipe	Warranty	Calibration/Meter Performance Check	Power Source	Memory
Glucometer M+ Bayer Corp. Diagnostics Division (800) 348-8100	5.5" × 3.2" × 1.0" 8.5 oz	Glucofilm test strips $37	Wipe: manual timing	3 years	Lot-specific code for each new vial; push button to select code; check "paddle" to confirm meter electronic performance	Nonreplace-able battery for memory; two AA batteries for LED screen	Stores up to 300 entries of test results and insulin, meal plan, exercise, and other events with date and time
MediSense 2 Pen Sensor **MediSense 2 Card Sensor** MediSense, Inc. (800) 527-3339	5.4" × 0.4" (1.1 oz) 3.7" × 2.2" × 0.4" 1.5 oz	MediSense 2 test strips $34-$37	Nonwipe; automatic timing	4 years	Calibrator packaged in each box of strips	Nonreplace-able batteries	Stores 10 test results
One Touch Basic LifeScan, Inc. (800) 227-8862	4.7" × 2.6" × 1.1" 4.8 oz	One Touch test strips $31	Nonwipe; automatic timing	3 years	Lot-specific code for each new vial; push button to select code; check strip to confirm meter electronic performance	J-cell battery	Stores previous test result

Product	Dimensions/Weight	Test strips	Timing	Warranty	Calibration	Battery	Memory
One Touch Profile LifeScan, Inc. (800) 227-8862	4.3" × 2.5" × 1.2" 4.5 oz	One Touch test strips $31	Nonwipe; automatic timing	5 years	Lot-specific code for each new vial; push button to select code; check to confirm meter electronic performance	Two AA alkaline batteries	Stores 250 test results with date, time, insulin dose, carbohydrates and events
Precision Q.I.D. MediSense, Inc. (800) 527-3339	3.8" × 1.9" × 0.6" 1.4 oz	Precision Q.I.D. test strips $32-$35	Nonwipe; automatic timing	4 years	Calibrator packaged in each box of strips	Nonreplaceable batteries	Stores 10 test results for visual feedback; capable of storing 125 test results for data management
Supreme Blood Glucose Monitor Hypoguard Ltd. (Distributed by Chronimed) (800) 876-6540	5.2" × 2.4" × 0.8" 4.8 oz	Supreme test strips $29	Nonwipe; automatic timing	2 years	Lot-specific code for each new vial; push button to select code	6-volt J-cell battery	Stores 14 test results

continued on next page ↓

10

Product	Dimensions/ Weight	Strip Name/ Price (50 strips)	Wipe/ Nonwipe	Warranty	Calibration/Meter Performance Check	Power Source	Memory
SureStep Lifescan, Inc. (800) 227-8862	3.5" × 2.4" × 0.8"	SureStep test strips $35	Nonwipe; automatic timing	3 years	Built-in button for coding; automatic internal diagnostics; no check strip required	Two AAA alkaline batteries	Stores 10 test results
Ultra+ Home Diagnostics, Inc. (800) 342-7226	3.5" × 2.5" × 0.5" 3.0 oz	Ultra+ test strips $30–$36	Nonwipe; automatic timing	2 years	Lot-specific code for each new vial; push button to select code; performs check strip automatically to confirm meter performance	J-cell battery	Stores 50 test results

Adapted from: Measuring the meters. *Diabetes Self-Management.* 1996;May/June:12-15.

TABLE 10.3 — MEASURING THE METERS: FEATURES

Product	Range* (mg/dL)	Visual Read Capability	Test Time (seconds)	Control Solution[†]	Hematocrit Range[‡]	Special Features
Accu-Chek Advantage Boehringer-Mannheim Corp. (800) 858-8072	10-60	No	40	Low and high levels	20-65% < 200 25-55% > 200	Error message for insufficient drop. No cleaning necessary. Data port for data management with Accu-Chek PDM Pro patient data management system. Temperature warning message.
Accu-Chek Easy Boehringer-Mannheim Corp. (800) 858-8072	20-500	Qualitative "ballpark" verification only	15-60	Normal level	30% - 55%	Rejects inadequate blood sample. Blood is supplied to absorbent test strip outside of the meter. 7-day average and 14-event codes. Data port for data management with Accu-Chek PDM Pro patient data management system.
Accu-Chek Instant Boehringer-Mannheim Corp. (800) 858-8072	20-500	Yes	12	Low and high levels	30% - 55%	Fast Flow test strip pad architecture is designed to spread the drop of blood quickly and evenly to minimize spills and ensure accurate results. Temperature warning symbol automatically tags values that are out of normal operating range.
Accu-Chek III Boehringer-Mannheim Corp. (800) 858-8072	20-500	Yes	120	Low and high levels	35% - 55%	Rejects inadequate sample. Displays time and date.

10

continued on next page ↓

Product	Range* (mg/dL)	Visual Read Capability	Test Time (seconds)	Control Solution[†]	Hematocrit Range[‡]	Special Features
Checkmate Plus Cascade Medical, Inc. (800) 525-6718	25-500	No	15-70	Low and high levels	20% - 55%	Automatic sample volume check. Built-in lancing device. Automatic calibration, temperature and hematocrit correction. Four alarms to remind user when to test. Memory of insulin type and dosage with time and date. Data port for data management with Check Link Diabetes Care Software.
Diascan Partner Home Diagnostics, Inc. (800) 342-7226	10-600	Yes (for verification by a sighted helper)	90	Low and high levels	20% - 60%	Audio blood glucose monitoring system for visually impaired persons. Voice module guides user through entire procedure. Three-setting volume control. Repeat message button. Earphone for private testing. Portable with shoulder strap carrying case. User can smear blood sample onto strip with accurate results.
Diascan-S Home Diagnostics, Inc. (800) 342-7226	10-600	Yes	90	Low and high levels	20% - 60%	User can smear blood sample onto strip with accurate results. Large display area. Temperature compensation.
Exactech Card Sensor MediSense, Inc. (800) 527-3339	40-450	No	30	Low and high levels	25% - 55%	Large display area. No cleaning required. Credit card size and shape.

Glucometer Elite Bayer Corp. Diagnostics Division (800) 348-8100	40-500	No	60	Normal level	20% - 60%	Provides memory and average. Option to delete control results from memory. Small blood sample required. Blood sample is drawn into test strip, not put on the test strip. No cleaning required. Turned on when test strip is inserted; no buttons.
Glucometer Encore Bayer Corp. Diagnostics Division (800) 348-8100	10-600	No	15-60	Normal level	20% - 60%	Option to delete control results from memory. Cleaning required.
Glucometer M+ Bayer Corp. Diagnostics Division (800) 348-8100	20-500	"Ballpark" verification only	60	Low, normal, and high levels	20% - 50%	Meter and logbook combined allows input of insulin, meal plan, exercise, and other events. 14-day average of results. Alarm clock functions. Connects with optional phone modem.
MediSense 2 Pen Sensor **MediSense 2 Card Sensor** MediSense, Inc. (800) 527-3339	20-600	No	20	Low and high levels	35% - 55%	**Pen:** Pen-size meter. **Card:** Credit-card size with large display area. No cleaning required. Automatic start. Data port for data management with Precision Link Blood Glucose Data Management System.
One Touch Basic LifeScan, Inc. (800) 227-8862	0-600	No	45	Normal level	25% - 60%	30-day money-back guarantee. Sensor indicates when there is not enough blood and when the meter must be cleaned. Spanish/English language choices. Strip area can be removed for cleaning.

10

continued on next page →

Product	Range* (mg/dL)	Visual Read Capability	Test Time (seconds)	Control Solution[†]	Hematocrit Range[‡]	Special Features
One Touch Profile LifeScan, Inc. (800) 227-8862	0-600	No	45	Normal level	25% -60%	30-day money-back guarantee. Includes record-keeping features regarding test results, insulin dosages, meals and other events. Displays 4-day and 30-day test averages. Multiple language choices. Error detection. Strip area can be removed for cleaning. Data port for data management with in Touch Diabetes Management software. Optional: Synthetic voice attachment connects to the meter and annunciates all messages.
Precision Q.I.D. MediSense, Inc. (800) 527-3339	20-500	No	20	Normal, low, and high levels	30% - 60%	Small blood sample required. Large display area. Can reapply blood sample within 30 seconds. Data port for data management with Precision Link.
Supreme Blood Glucose Monitor Hypoguard Ltd. (Distributed by Chronimed) (800) 876-6540	40-400	Yes	< 50	Low and high levels	35% - 55%	Blood sample is applied to the strip, which is then inserted into the meter. Strip carrier can be removed for cleaning. 30-day money-back guarantee.

	0-500	Yes	15 seconds minimum; 30 seconds average	Normal level	25% - 60%	Blue confirmation dot ensures adequate sample size. Absorbent test strip stays dry to the touch. Can drop or dab blood on strip. Large universal symbols guide users.
SureStep Lifescan, Inc. (800) 227-8862						
Ultra+ Home Diagnostics, Inc. (800) 342-7226	0-600	"Ballpark" verification only	45	Low, medium, and high levels	30% - 55%	Large display area. Automatic temperature compensation.

*Blood glucose range.

†Control solution is a liquid that contains a known amount of glucose that can be used to verify that a new package of strips is working properly with the meter.

‡Hematocrit range refers to the percentage of total blood that consists of red blood cells. If the pateint has a medical condition, such as anemia, that affects the percentage of red blood cells and hematocrit is not within the range that the meter reads, the results may be inaccurate.

Adapted from: Measuring the meters. *Diabetes Self-Management.* 1996;May/June:12-15.

- Prebreakfast — four to seven tests per week
- Prelunch — two to three tests per week
- 2 hours postdinner — two to three tests per week.

Patients in this category generally require one to three tests per day when SMCBG values are consistent. Patients can make nonpharmacologic changes in their diabetic regimen depending on the results (Table 10.4).

SMCBG for Patients Who Take Insulin

SMCBG is critical for all patients who take exogenous insulin, particularly those on intensive insulin regimens or on combination therapy. The type of insulin regimen used should dictate the frequency of

---

TABLE 10.4 — TECHNIQUES USED TO ADJUST FOR PREMEAL HYPERGLYCEMIA

Nonpharmacologic
- Increase the time interval between insulin injection and consumption of the meal.
- Consume less than the usual amount of calories.
- Eliminate or replace foods containing refined carbohydrates or that have a high glycemic index, such as fruit exchanges.
- Spread the calories over an extended period of time.
- Exercise lightly after a meal.

Pharmacologic
- Increase the amount of fast-acting insulin via an algorithm.
- Make the appropriate long-term adjustment in insulin dose to prevent hyperglycemia at a particular time if a consistent trend is identified.

Source: Edelman SV, Henry RR. Insulin therapy for normalizing glycosylated hemoglobin in type II diabetes: application, benefits, and risks. *Diabetes Reviews*. 1994;3:310.

SMCBG, with attention to insulin pharmacokinetics and the timing of insulin injections. The best time to evaluate the effectiveness of a dose is at the peak time of action of a particular type of insulin (see Table 8.1).

Frequent SMCBG is necessary to fine-tune an insulin regimen to the needs and responses of a given patient. Ideally, SMCBG should be performed 4 to 6 times per day (before each meal, at bedtime, and occasionally at 3:00 AM, which is the approximate time of early morning glucose nadir). A more intensive SMCBG schedule would be a pre- and 2-hour postprandial measurement and at bedtime, depending on the frequency of insulin doses.

SMCBG recommendations for patients on insulin therapy:

- One injection per day — two tests per day, no less than one to three depending on metabolic control.
- Two injections per day — four tests per day (before each meal and at bedtime)
- Intensive regimen (multiple injections, external pumps) — four to seven tests per day.

10

Results should be recorded in a log book that is brought to each office visit so the physician can evaluate the effectiveness of the insulin regimen and determine the most appropriate insulin dosage adjustments (Figure 10.1). Selected patients should be instructed to apply their SMCBG results as the data become available. Making immediate dosage adjustments based on SMCBG feedback is evidence of the true benefit of this self-assessment tool. Additionally, some meter logs can be downloaded directly to a personal computer.

When SMCBG reveals premeal hyperglycemia, a number of different methods can be used in addition to adjusting the dose of insulin to reduce daily glycemic excursions (Table 10.4).

FIGURE 10.1 — WEEKLY SELF-MONITORING BLOOD GLUCOSE RECORD SHEET

Name _____   SSI #: _____ – _____ – _____

Address _____   Home PH#: (___) ___ – ___

City _____   Work PH#: (___) ___ – ___

State _____ Zip _____ – ___   Fax #: (___) ___ – ___

                                        Pager #: (___) ___ – ___

INSTRUCTIONS: Record time of day in upper box and glucose readings in lower box.

Day/Date (m/d/y)	AM Breakfast		AM INSULIN	Noon	PM Dinner		PM INSULIN	Comments
	Before	After			Before	After		
SUNDAY ___/___/___								
MONDAY ___/___/___								
TUESDAY ___/___/___								

130

						Weekly Averages
WEDNESDAY __/__/__						
THURSDAY __/__/__						
FRIDAY __/__/__						
SATURDAY __/__/__						

Daily Averages

	SUNDAY	MONDAY	TUESDAY	WEDNESDAY	THURSDAY	FRIDAY	SATURDAY	Weekly Averages
TIMES OF DAY								
GLUCOSE READINGS								
WEIGHT								

TOTAL UNITS FOR THE WEEK: AM _____ + PM _____ =

10

FIGURE 10.2 — ALGORITHM FORM USED FOR PATIENTS ON INTENSIVE INSULIN THERAPY

Name_____

Provider_____

Date_____

Phone_____

Time between injection and meal (min)		Blood glucose value (mg/dL)	Breakfast	Lunch	Dinner	Bedtime	Bedtime snack size
Humalog	Regular						
0	5-15	< 80					large
5	30	81-150					medium
5-15	30-45	151-200					small
15-30	45-60	201-250					none
30	60	251-300					none
30+	60+	301-350					none
30+	60+	351-400					none
30+	60+	401-450					none
30+	60+	451+					none

AM long-acting insulin dose_____

PM long-acting insulin dose_____

☐ Take before dinner   ☐ Take at bedtime

As the premeal blood glucose value increases, the amount of regular insulin recommended also increases and is adjusted based on postprandial glucose values. The time between the insulin injection and the meal also should be increased as the premeal blood glucose values increase, thus improving postprandial glucose values. If the patient consistently requires higher regular insulin doses at a particular time (3 consecutive days), appropriate long-term adjustments should be made.

Source: VA Endocrinology Clinic, VA Hospital, UCSD, La Jolla, California.

10

Applying SMCBG Results to Adjust Insulin Doses

Patients can be taught how to analyze and use SMCBG data to effectively make adjustments in their insulin doses so that they can maintain and improve glycemic control. Insulin algorithms can be used with SMCBG to make appropriate day-to-day changes in insulin dosing and to guide long-term treatment. The insulin algorithm shown in Figure 10.2 is used for patients receiving intensive insulin therapy. Self-adjustment guidelines for patients on a split-mixed regimen are shown in Table 10.5; insulin unit changes are provided by the physician on an individualized basis.

REFERENCES

1. American Diabetes Association. *Medical Management of Non–insulin-dependent (Type II) Diabetes*, 3rd ed. Alexandria, Va: American Diabetes Association; 1994:52-54.

2. Davidson MB. *Diabetes Mellitus: Diagnosis and Treatment*, 3rd ed. New York: Churchill Livingstone; 1991:213-291.

3. American Diabetes Association. Consensus statement: self-monitoring of blood glucose. Clinical practice recommendations 1995. *Diabetes Care*. 1995;18(suppl 1):47-52.

4. The Diabetes Control and Complications Trial Research Group. The effect of intensive treatment of diabetes on the development and progression of long-term complications in insulin-dependent diabetes mellitus. *N Engl J Med*. 1993;329: 977-986.

5. Peragallo-Dittko V, ed. *A Core Curriculum for Diabetes Education*, 2nd ed. Chicago: American Association of Diabetes Educators; 1993:259-279.

TABLE 10.5 — PATIENT SELF ADJUSTMENT OF INSULIN DOSAGE, SPLIT-MIXED REGIMEN

1. If the prebreakfast blood sugar is greater than 140 mg/dL for 3 days in a row, then increase the evening NPH dosage by ____ units.

2. If the prelunch blood sugar is greater than 150 mg/dL for 3 days in a row, then increase the morning regular insulin dosage by ____ units.

3. If the predinner blood sugar is greater than 150 mg/dL for 3 days in a row, then increase the morning NPH insulin dosage by ____ units.

4. If the bedtime blood sugar is greater than 180 mg/dL for 3 days in a row, then increase the predinner regular insulin dosage by ____ units.

5. If the prebreakfast blood sugar is less than 100 mg/dL for 3 days in a row, then decrease the evening NPH insulin dosage by ____ units.

6. If the prelunch blood sugar is less than 100 mg/dL for 3 days in a row, then decrease the morning regular insulin dosage by ____ units.

7. If the predinner blood sugar is less than 100 mg/dL for 3 days in a row, then decrease the morning NPH insulin dosage by ____ units.

8. If the bedtime blood sugar is less than 100 mg/dL for 3 days in a row, then decrease the predinner regular insulin dosage by ____ units.

9. If more than one change in insulin dosage is needed, adjust the NPH dosage first before making any changes in the regular dosage.

10. Remember not to make changes in the insulin dosage more frequently than every 3 days, and do not hesitate to call me for any questions at (____)____-____.

10

_____
Physician/Caregiver

Source: VA Endocrinology Clinic, VA Hospital, UCSD, La Jolla, California.

Additional Reading

Fleming DR. Accuracy of blood glucose monitoring for patients: what it is and how to achieve it. *Diabetes Educ*. 1994;20:495-500.

Greyson J. Quality control in patient self-monitoring of blood glucose. *Diabetes Care*. 1993;16:1306-1308.

Harris MI, Cowie CC, Howie LJ. Self-monitoring of blood glucose by adults with diabetes in the Unites States population. *Diabetes Care*. 1993;16:1116-1123.

Nettles A. User error in blood glucose monitoring. The National Steering Committee for Quality Assurance report. *Diabetes Care*. 1993;16:946-948.

11   Acute Complications

Patients with type II diabetes are prone to developing acute complications such as:
- Metabolic
  - Diabetic ketoacidosis (DKA)
  - Hyperosmolar hyperglycemic nonketotic syndrome (HHNS)
  - Hypoglycemia
- Infection (poor wound healing)
- Quality of life
  - Nocturia
  - Poor sleep
  - Daytime tiredness
  - Tooth and gum disease
  - Cognitive impairment.

The most common acute complications of diabetes are metabolic problems (DKA, HHNS, hypoglycemia) and infection. In addition, the quality of life of patients with chronic and severe hypoglycemia is adversely affected. Characteristic symptoms of tiredness and lethargy can become severe and lead to increased falls in the elderly, decreased school performance in children, and decreased work performance in adults.

Metabolic

■ Diabetic Ketoacidosis
This acute metabolic complication typically results from a profound insulin deficiency (absolute or relative) associated with uncontrolled type I diabetes mellitus and occasionally in decompensated type II diabetes.

Individuals with type II diabetes may develop DKA under certain conditions:

- Poor nutrition that contributes to dehydration and catabolism of fat to provide necessary calories
- Severe physiologic stress (eg, infection, myocardial infarction) that leads to increased levels of counterregulatory hormones (eg, epinephrine, cortisol, and glucagon), which stimulate beta-oxidation of fatty acids
- Chronic poor metabolic control that leads to decreased insulin secretion and decreased glucose uptake (glucose toxicity)
- Dehydration that leads to decreased excretion of ketones in urine and a buildup of ketone bodies in the blood.

Key characteristics include:[1]

- Hyperglycemia (300 to 800 mg/dL although usually < 600 mg/dL, concentration not related to severity of DKA)
- Ketosis (pH 6.8 to 7.3) and acidosis (HCO_3, 0 to 15 mEq/L)
- Dehydration caused by:
  – Nausea
  – Vomiting
  – The consequent inadequate oral intake
- Electrolyte depletion (eg, potassium, magnesium).

Precipitating factors vary from individual to individual and may include the following (approximately 50% of which are preventable):

- Illness and infection; increased production of glucocorticoids by adrenal gland promotes gluconeogenesis; increased production of epinephrine and norepinephrine increases glycogenolysis

- Inadequate insulin dosage due to omission or reduction of doses by patient, physician, or clinic; patients with GI distress often decrease or eliminate their insulin doses thinking that less insulin is needed when food intake is decreased; this practice can be dangerous because GI symptoms are key features of DKA
- Initial manifestation of type I diabetes in the elderly misdiagnosed as type II diabetes
- Chronic untreated hyperglycemia (glucose toxicity).

Pathophysiology of DKA

Diabetic ketoacidosis is a metabolic acidosis caused by a significant insulin deficiency. The following physiologic abnormalities are characteristic of DKA and require prompt correction:
- Chronic hyperglycemia and glucose toxicity
- Acidosis caused by catabolism of fat and the buildup of ketone bodies
- Low blood volume because of dehydration (loss of fluid and electrolytes)
- Hyperosmolality because of renal water loss and water depletion from sweating, nausea, and vomiting; and associated potassium loss.

11

Symptoms and Signs of DKA

The symptoms and signs of DKA are shown in Table 11.1. These are classic for DKA in type I diabetes, although they are never as severe in patients with type II diabetes. Polyuria and polydipsia are symptoms of osmotic diuresis secondary to hyperglycemia. Nonspecific symptoms include weakness, lethargy, headache, and myalgia; specific symptoms of DKA are gastrointestinal and respiratory. The GI symptoms probably are related to the ketosis and/or acidosis. The chief respiratory complaint of dyspnea actually is an inability to catch one's breath. This type of hyperven-

TABLE 11.1 — SYMPTOMS AND SIGNS OF CLASSIC DKA

Symptoms of DKA
- Nausea
- Vomiting
- Abdominal pain
- Dyspnea
- Myalgia
- Headache
- Anorexia
- Characteristic symptoms of hyperglycemia

Signs of DKA
- Hypothermia
- Hyperpnea (Kussmaul's respiration)
- Acetone breath
- "Dehydration" (intravascular volume depletion)
- Hyporeflexia
- "Acute abdomen" (tenderness to palpation, muscle guarding, diminished bowel sounds)
- Stupor (mild to frank coma)
- Hypotonia
- Uncoordinated ocular movements
- Fixed, dilated pupils

Source: Davidson MB. *Diabetes Mellitus: Diagnosis and Treatment*, 3rd ed. New York: Churchill Livingstone; 1991.

tilation unrelated to exertion is the ventilatory response to metabolic acidosis termed Kussmaul's respiration.

Because the signs are not specific to DKA, physicians should be alert to a constellation of evidence that points to the possibility of DKA.

Because other diseases and conditions may mimic DKA and precipitate and/or coexist with DKA, the following differential diagnoses (and representative DKA symptoms) should be considered:

- Cerebrovascular accident (altered mental status)
- Brainstem hemorrhage (hyperventilation, glucosuria)

- Hypoglycemia (altered mental status, tachycardia)
- Metabolic acidosis (hyperventilation, anion gap acidosis):
  - Uremia
  - Salicylates
  - Methanol
  - Ethylene glycol
- Gastroenteritis (nausea, vomiting, abdominal pain)
- Pneumonia (hyperventilation).

Laboratory Evaluation
Initial laboratory values are shown in Table 11.2.

Treatment
Although aggressive therapy is not usually necessary in type II diabetes, the following treatment strategies are for severe cases and for true type I diabetes misdiagnosed as type II diabetes because of the patient's age at presentation. The goals of treatment are to:
- Correct fluid and electrolyte disturbances
- Restore and maintain normal glucose metabolism
- Correct acidosis.

The cornerstones of DKA therapy are administering fluids and insulin immediately. Potassium and phosphate replacement, and bicarbonate therapy also may be necessary for certain patients, depending on the severity of the DKA. This is rarely the case in patients with type II diabetes. The following treatment guidelines provide an overview for managing DKA.[1] It is not unusual that patients with type II diabetes can be treated adequately in a general hospital ward and not in an intensive care unit.

Fluid and Electrolyte Replacement
- Based on the degree of dehydration and the patient's cardiovascular status.

141

TABLE 11.2 — INITIAL LABORATORY VALUES FOR PATIENTS EXPERIENCING DKA

Test	Result	Remarks
Glucose	300-800 mg/dL	Concentrations not related to severity of DKA
Ketone bodies	Strong at least in undiluted plasma	Measures only acetoacetate, not β-hydroxybutyrate
[HCO_3]	0-15 mEq/L	Concentrations related to severity of DKA
pH	6.8-7.3	Concentrations related to severity of DKA
[K]	Low, normal, or high	Total body depletion; heart responsive to extracellular concentration
Phosphate	Usually normal or slightly elevated; occasionally slightly low	Associated with phosphaturia; marked decrease with treatment in levels of both serum and urine phosphates
Creatine/BUN	Usually mildly increased	May be prerenal; spurious increases in creatinine by acetoacetate in some automated methods
WBC count	Usually increased	Possibility of leukemoid reaction (even in absence of infection)

Amylase	Often increased	Predominant form of salivary gland origin
Hemoglobin, hematocrit, total protein	Often increased	Secondary to contracted plasma volume
AST, ALT, LDH	Can be mildly elevated	Spurious increases in transaminases due to acetoacetate interference in older colorimetric methods

Abbreviations: HCO_3, concentration of bicarbonate; K, concentration of potassium; BUN, blood urea nitrogen; WBC, white blood cell; AST, aspartate aminotransferase; ALT, alanine aminotransferase; LDH, lactic dehydrogenase.

Source: Reprinted with permission from Davidson MB. *Diabetes Mellitus: Diagnosis and Treatment*, 3rd ed. New York: Churchill Livingstone; 1991:183.

- Also plays a critical role in lowering glucose concentrations; hyperglycemia will continue despite appropriate insulin therapy if hydration is not adequate.
- Oral hydration with a sodium-containing fluid is appropriate for a patient with mild DKA who is not vomiting.
- Most adults require IV fluid administration with normal (0.9%) or half-normal (0.45%) saline (normal saline should be used when intravascular volume depletion is extreme and half-normal saline when plasma volume contraction is more moderate).
- One liter of fluid should be given per hour for the first 2 hours; the rate can be decreased to 500 mL per hour when signs of intravascular volume depletion have subsided.
- IV fluids are continued until intravascular volume has been fully restored, as indicated by normal filling of neck veins or when the patient can tolerate fluids.

Insulin Therapy
- Most patients with type II diabetes can be treated successfully with frequent (every 3 to 4 hours) injections of regular insulin subcutaneously (5 to 15 units).
- A low dose of regular insulin can be administered via IV infusion at a rate of approximately 5 units per hour.
- If a 10% decrease in glucose concentration from the initial level is not observed after 2 hours, the infusion rate should be doubled to 10 units per hour.
- The insulin infusion can be discontinued and intermediate-acting NPH insulin can be started when HCO_3 is > 15 mEq/L and the patient can drink and eat light foods.

Potassium Replacement

- Usually is necessary after fluid and insulin therapy have been started because all modes of therapy reduce the serum [K].
- The goal is to maintain the serum [K] within the normal range.
- An ECG should be done as soon as possible. Potassium replacement is withheld if the patient is anuric or if the T waves are abnormally tall and peaked or have a high-normal configuration. If the T waves are normal, 20 mEq of potassium (with appropriate anion) is added to the first liter of replacement fluid. Low or flat T waves require the addition of 40 mEq of potassium.
- An ECG should be taken every 1 to 2 hours to evaluate treatment and adjust the potassium replacement regimen. Patients who are able to eat can receive potassium orally via food intake or potassium supplementation (12 to 15 mEq 3 times daily with meals).

Phosphate Replacement

- Phosphate levels should be measured initially; some physicians use potassium phosphate for replacement if PO_4 is in the low or low-normal range.

Bicarbonate Therapy

- Not necessary for most patients but may be considered under certain circumstances, such as for patients with life-threatening hyperkalemia, lactic acidosis, or severe acidosis (pH < 7.2) with shock that does not respond to fluid replacement.
- When necessary, bicarbonate should be added to 0.45% saline and infused slowly over at least 1

hour; it should never be given in an IV bolus because of the risk of death secondary to hypokalemia.

Glucose concentrations decreased by about 75 to 100 mg/dL/h with low-dose insulin infusion, reaching levels of 200 to 300 mg/dL within 4 to 5 hours. Dextrose generally is added to the infusion at this point in therapy to avoid hypoglycemia from continued insulin administration, which still is necessary to treat ketosis and acidosis. Approximately 12 to 24 hours of treatment is necessary to reverse ketosis for most patients; some patients may have ketone bodies for several days.

■ Hyperosmolar Hyperglycemic Nonketotic Syndrome

This acute metabolic complication is a life-threatening crisis with a high mortality rate that usually is seen in:

- Elderly patients with type II diabetes (particularly those in nursing homes without free access to water)
- People with undiagnosed diabetes
- Those with diabetes that is diagnosed after a long period of uncontrolled hyperglycemia.

Pathophysiology of HHNS

Hyperosmolar hyperglycemic nonketotic syndrome has four key clinical features:

- Severe hyperglycemia—blood glucose usually > 600 mg/dL (> 33.3 mM) and generally 1000 mg/dL to 2000 mg/dL (55.5 mM to111.1 mM)
- Absence of or slight ketosis
- Plasma or serum hyperosmolality (> 340 mOsm)
- Profound dehydration.

In clinical practice, patients often are seen who have these characteristics but also have mild ketosis and acidosis. Although HHNS and DKA represent opposite ends of a continuum, many patients have some aspects of each syndrome. The two conditions have a similar pathophysiology, clinical signs and symptoms, and treatments, with certain important exceptions.

Symptoms and Signs of HHNS

Patients typically develop excessive thirst, confusion, and physical signs of severe dehydration. A comparison of the key features of HHNS and DKA is shown in Table 11.3; several important differences exist in the symptoms and signs:

- Gastrointestinal (GI) symptoms usually are milder in HHNS than in DKA in the absence of ketosis and acidosis. Because of a lack of severe GI problems (which prompted patients with DKA to seek medical attention within 1 to 2 days), patients with HHNS may tolerate polyuria and polydipsia for weeks and consequently lose significant quantities of fluids and electrolytes before seeking help. Average fluid loss in HHNS is 9 L vs 6.5 L in DKA.
- Kussmaul's respiration is rarely observed because of a lack of severe acidosis.
- Decreased mentation (mild confusion, lethargy) and lack of normal responsiveness are common and correlate best with serum osmolality. These are the usual reasons that patients with HHNS seek medical attention.
- Focal neurologic signs may be present and may mimic a cerebrovascular event (hemisensory deficits, hemiparesis, aphasia, seizures); these signs decline as biochemical status returns to normal.

11

TABLE 11.3 — DIABETIC KETOACIDOSIS AND HYPERGLYCEMIC HYPEROSMOLAR NONKETOTIC SYNDROME: COMPARISON OF SOME SALIENT FEATURES

Feature	Conditions	
	DKA	HHNS
Age of patients	Usually < 40 years	Usually > 60 years
Duration of symptoms	Usually < 2 days	Usually > 5 days
Glucose level	Usually < 600 mg/dL (< 33.3 mmol/L)	Usually > 800 mg/dL (> 44.4 mmol/L)
Sodium concentration	More likely to be normal, or low	More likely to be normal or high
Potassium concentration	High, normal or low	High, normal, or low
Bicarbonate concentration	Low	Normal
Ketone bodies	At least 4+ in 1:1 dilution	< 2+ in 1:1 dilution

pH	Low	Low
Serum osmolality	Usually < 350 mOsm/kg (< 350 mmol/kg)	Usually > 350 mOsm/kg (> 350 mmol/kg)
Cerebral edema	Often subclinical; occasionally clinical	Subclinical has not been evaluated; rarely clinical
Prognosis	3% to 10% mortality	10% to 20% mortality
Subsequent course	Insulin therapy required in virtually all cases	Insulin therapy not required in many cases

Abbreviations: DKA, diabetic ketoacidosis; HHNS, hyperglycemic hyperosmolar nonketotic syndrome.

Source: Reprinted with permission from Peragallo-Dittko V, ed. *A Core Curriculum for Diabetes Education*, 2nd ed. Chicago: American Association of Diabetes Educators; 1993:326.

11

A diagnosis of HHNS usually is made easily if one has a high index of suspicion. Patients may be admitted to the neurology or neurosurgical service because only neurologic conditions are considered initially. Routine urine and blood tests can help clarify the diagnosis of HHNS. Health-care professionals need to be alert for signs of HHNS in patients at chronic-care facilities because this diagnosis tends to be overlooked in such settings.

Laboratory Evaluation

Typical laboratory values in HHNS are shown in Table 11.3.

Treatment

Life-saving measures may be needed immediately. The primary treatment goal is rehydration to restore circulating plasma volume and correct electrolyte deficits. In addition, the precipitating event should be identified and corrected, and other goals similar to those described for treatment of DKA should be instituted, including providing adequate insulin to restore and maintain normal glucose metabolism. Glucose concentration is the only biochemical end point because patients with HHNS do not have ketosis or acidosis.

- Cardiovascular status should be monitored closely and frequently during fluid replacement to avoid precipitating congestive heart failure, given the fact that most patients with HHNS are older and have preexisting heart disease.
- Insulin is administered in the same manner as for patients with DKA. At glucose concentrations of 250 mg/dL, the rate of insulin infusion should be decreased to 2 to 3 U/h and dextrose should be added to the IV fluid because oral intake will not be possible for many hours to a few days.

- Dextrose (50 g) should be given intravenously every 8 hours and insulin dose adjusted accordingly (decreased 1 to 3 U/h) based on plasma glucose measurements every 4 hours.
- Potassium replacement follows the same guidelines as for DKA, with consideration of the special conditions of patients with HHNS (underlying renal disease is associated with lower urinary potassium losses, preexisting heart disease is associated with greater susceptibility to the effects of potassium).
- Bicarbonate therapy is contraindicated.
- Phosphate replacement follows the same guidelines as for DKA, with consideration of the effect of phosphate on underlying renal disease.

■ Hypoglycemia

This metabolic problem occurs in both type I and type II diabetes when there is an imbalance between food intake and the appropriate dosage and timing of drug therapy (oral agents, insulin). Other factors that contribute to hypoglycemia are:

- Exercise
- Alcohol intake
- Other drugs
- Decreased liver or kidney function.

Signs of Hypoglycemia

The incidence of hypoglycemia in patients with type II diabetes is several orders of magnitude lower than in type I diabetes. Nonetheless, patients taking insulin and/or sulfonylureas are prone to hypoglycemia.

Hypoglycemia should be suspected in patients who demonstrate the following clinical signs;[2] a diagnosis of hypoglycemia is confirmed in a symptomatic patient if a plasma glucose level < 60 mg/dL (< 3.3 mM) is found:

- Mild hypoglycemia is associated with adrenergic or cholinergic symptoms such as:
  - Pallor
  - Diaphoresis
  - Tachycardia
  - Palpitations
  - Hunger
  - Paresthesias
  - Shakiness
- Moderate hypoglycemia is associated with neuroglycopenic symptoms of altered mental and/or neurologic functioning such as:
  - Inability to concentrate
  - Confusion
  - Slurred speech
  - Irrational or uncontrolled behavior
  - Slowed reaction time
  - Blurred vision
  - Somnolence
  - Extreme fatigue
- Severe hypoglycemia is associated with extreme impairment of neurologic function to the extent that the assistance of another person is needed to obtain treatment; symptoms include:
  - Completely automatic/disoriented behavior
  - Loss of consciousness
  - Inability to arouse from sleep
  - Seizures.

  Nocturnal hypoglycemia is associated with over 50% of cases of severe hypoglycemia;[2] early symptoms do not awaken patients and the predinner intermediate-acting insulins may cause hyperinsulinemia in the early morning hours.

It is important to understand that hypoglycemia does not necessarily progress in a linear fashion from mild to severe. For example, some patients might develop neuroglycopenic symptoms before adrenergic or cholinergic symptoms, and other patients may overlook or ignore adrenergic or cholinergic symptoms and progress to neuroglycopenia.

Treatment

The goal of treatment is to normalize the plasma glucose level as quickly as possible.

- Mild hypoglycemia is treated most effectively by having the patient ingest approximately 15 g of carbohydrate by mouth. Sources of carbohydrate (15 g)[2] include:
  - 3 glucose tablets (5 g each)
  - $1/2$ cup fruit juice
  - 2 tablespoons raisins
  - 5 Lifesavers® candy
  - $1/2$ to $3/4$ cup regular soda (not diet)
  - 1 cup milk

  If symptoms continue, treatment may need to be repeated in 15 minutes. Most patients can resume normal activity following treatment.
- For moderate hypoglycemia, larger amounts of carbohydrate (15 to 30 g) that are rapidly absorbed may be needed. Patients usually are instructed to consume additional food after the initial treatment and wait approximately 30 minutes until resuming activity. Measuring blood glucose levels during treatment and the recovery periods can help determine the effectiveness of treatment. Some patients, however, may continue to have neuroglycopenic symptoms for an hour or longer after blood glucose levels have increased to above 100 mg/dL.
- Severe hypoglycemia requires rapid treatment. IV glucose (50 cc 50% dextrose or glucose followed by 10% dextrose drip) is the most effective route; however, glucagon (1 mg for adults) can be administered at home with positive re-

11

sults. Individuals who are unable to swallow should be given glucose gel, honey, syrup, or jelly on the inside of the cheek. After the inital response, a rapid-acting, carbohydrate-containing liquid should be given until nausea subsides; then a small snack or meal can be consumed. Blood glucose levels should be monitored frequently for several hours to assure that the levels remain normal and to avoid overtreatment. The individual's health-care team should be informed of any severe hypoglycemic episodes.

Prevention

Patients can take certain measures to avoid hypoglycemia:

- Know the signs and symptoms of hypoglycemia.
- Try to eat meals on a regular schedule.
- Carry a source of carbohydrate (at least 10 to 15 g).
- Perform SMCBG regularly for early detection of low blood glucose levels; initiate treatment at the first signs of hypoglycemia.
- Use regular insulin 30 minutes before eating. (Patients who take their regular insulin immediately before or after the meal will be prone to delayed hypoglycemia.)
- Schedule exercise appropriately; adjust meal times, calorie intake, or insulin dosing to accommodate physical activity; use SMCBG (before, during, after strenuous activity) to determine the effect of exercise on blood glucose levels and to detect low blood glucose levels.
- Check blood glucose level before going to sleep to avoid nocturnal hypoglycemia; perform nocturnal (3:00 AM) monitoring:
  - If hypoglycemia has occurred during the night
  - When evening insulin has been adjusted

- When strenuous activity has occurred the previous day
- During times of irregular eating schedules or erratic glucose control.

Infection

Infection is the primary cause of metabolic abnormalities leading to diabetic coma in patients with diabetes. Because of the potentially severe consequences of untreated infections, prompt diagnosis and treatment is essential. Common infections in patients with diabetes are shown in Table 11.4.

Quality of Life

Patients with blood glucose values consistently greater than 200 mg/dL will have a reduced quality of life. Poorly controlled blood glucose values will lead to excessive thirst and urination, causing nocturia and poor sleep. Poor sleep will lead to daytime tiredness and poor work performance in adults. Patients will have frequent urinary tract infections, tooth and gum disease and blurry vision. It has also been shown that the elderly experience cognitive impairment and a higher incidence of falls.

REFERENCES

1. Davidson MB. *Diabetes Mellitus: Diagnosis and Treatment*, 3rd ed. New York: Churchill Livingstone; 1991.

2. Peragallo-Dittko V, ed. *A Core Curriculum for Diabetes Education*, 2nd ed. Chicago: American Association of Diabetes Educators; 1993.

TABLE 11.4 — INFECTIONS COMMON OR SPECIAL TO PATIENTS WITH DIABETES MELLITUS	
Type of Infection	**Comments**
Cutaneous Furunculosis Carbuncles	For reasons not clear, patients with diabetes mellitus may be prone to recurrent furunculosis and carbuncles. Unless vascular insufficiency is present, warm compresses may be used for treatment.
Vulvovaginitis (less frequently, scrotal infections)	*Candida* skin infection commonly occurs in warm, moist areas, particularly in the region of the genitalia (also on the inner thighs and under the breasts). This is particularly common in people with type II diabetes who are overweight or who have been taking antibiotics. These infections can cause extreme discomfort to the patient and result in breakdown of skin, which may allow entry of more virulent organisms. Good glycemic control and local supportive antifungal treatment usually will resolve the problem.
Cellulitis, alone or in combination with lower extremity vascular ulcers	To prevent the spread of infection to bone and the necessity of amputation, treatment of infected ulcers and surrounding cellulitis must be aggressive. Antibiotics effective against bacteria recovered from the site (both aerobes and anaerobes should be expected) should be used, as well as surgical debridement and drainage.

Urinary tract	Asymptomatic bacteriuria occurs in up to 20% of patients with diabetes mellitus; some suggest that it be treated. Certainly, a patient with neurogenic bladder is susceptible to urinary tract infection and sepsis. Treatment is mandatory in patients with pyelonephritis. Patients with serious urinary tract infections should be hospitalized, the offending pathogens identified, and appropriate susceptibility tests performed.
Ear	Malignant external otitis is relatively rare, but when it occurs, it is most often seen in elderly diabetic patients with chronically draining ear and sudden onset of severe pain. *Pseudomonas aeruginosa* is the usual pathogenic organism. This condition is fatal in ~50% of cases. Immediate treatment should include appropriate antibiotic therapy and surgical debridement when indicated.

Source: Reprinted with permission from American Diabetes Association. *Medical Management of Non-insulin-dependent (Type II) Diabetes*, 3rd ed. Alexandria, Va: American Diabetes Association; 1994:81.

11

12 Long-term Complications

The long-term complications that may develop in patients with type II diabetes include:

- Macrovascular disease
  - Hypertension
  - Dyslipidemia
  - Myocardial infarction
  - Stroke
- Microvascular complications
  - Diabetic retinopathy
  - Diabetic nephropathy
  - Diabetic neuropathy
  - Diabetic diarrhea
  - Neurogenic bladder
  - Impaired cardiovascular reflexes
  - Sexual dysfunction
- Diabetic foot disorders.

The long-term, chronic complications of diabetes have the greatest impact on the health of individuals with diabetes as well as on the health-care system. Diabetes and its associated vascular complications are the fourth leading cause of death in the United States.[1] Consequently, early detection and aggressive treatment of these complications are essential to reduce associated morbidity and mortality. Striving for tight metabolic control also has been proven to help delay the onset and prevent the development of microvascular complications (diabetic retinopathy, nephropathy, and neuropathy).[2-3]

The Diabetes Control and Complications Trial (DCCT),[3] a multicenter, randomized clinical trial, investigated the effects of intensive therapy versus traditional therapy on the development and progression of vascular and neurologic complications of type I diabetes mellitus. The aim of intensive therapy was to achieve and maintain near-normal blood glucose values following a regimen of three or more daily insulin injections or treatment with an insulin pump. In contrast, only one or two insulin injections were used in conventional therapy. Patients were followed for a mean of 6.5 years and assessed regularly for the presence or progression of retinopathy, nephropathy, and neuropathy.

Intensive therapy proved to be highly effective in delaying the onset and slowing the progression of the long-term complications being evaluated in patients with type I diabetes. Furthermore, because hyperglycemia is associated with the development and progression of the same long-term complications in type II diabetes as in type I diabetes, the DCCT research group recommended extending the benefits of improved glycemic control to patients with type II diabetes. In response to the DCCT findings, the American Diabetes Association recommended striving for the best possible glycemic control in patients with type II diabetes, with the following goals: fasting and preprandial blood glucose level of 80 mg/dL to 120 mg/dL, bedtime or evening glucose level of 100 mg/dL to 140 mg/dL, and glycosylated hemoglobin of < 7% (normal reference range = 4% to 6%) or three standard deviations from the mean of the normal range.[4-5] Attempts to normalize glycemia and glycosylated hemoglobin should be balanced, however, with minimizing weight gain and hypoglycemia, and maintaining an acceptable quality of life.[5]

Macrovascular Disease

The incidence of the three major macrovascular diseases (coronary artery, cerebrovascular, and peripheral vascular) is greater in individuals with diabetes than in nondiabetic individuals, accounting for 80% of mortality in adults with diabetes. Atherosclerosis develops at an earlier age, accelerates more rapidly, and is more extensive in patients with diabetes than in nondiabetics matched by age, weight, and sex.

Type II diabetes is a risk factor for macrovascular disease as are conditions that commonly coexist in patients with diabetes (hypertension, dyslipidemia, and central obesity). Smoking and lack of exercise contribute to an increased risk in both type II diabetes and the nondiabetic population. In addition, renal insufficiency can increase the risk of macrovascular disease in diabetic individuals with microalbuminuria or gross proteinuria.

Weight control and exercise are safe and effective methods for modifying macrovascular risk and should form the basis to which all other treatments are added. The following treatments for hypertension and dyslipidemia should be applied where appropriate.

■ Hypertension

Hypertension should be treated vigorously in all patients with diabetes to limit and/or prevent the development and progression of atherosclerosis, nephropathy, and retinopathy. Lowering elevated blood pressure is the most important and immediate consideration, with a therapeutic goal of < 130/85 mm Hg. The goal for patients with isolated systolic hypertension (180 mm Hg) is 160 mm Hg; further reductions to 140 mm Hg are suggested if the treatment is well tolerated. The goal for patients with renal insufficiency should be < 120/80 mm Hg with a mean blood pressure < 93 mm Hg.

Treatment should be initiated with a no-added salt diet and weight loss (for obese patients) combined with appropriate aerobic exercise. Because patients with diabetes can be uniquely impacted by certain side effects of antihypertensives, physicians must be familiar with the potential complications of the classes of antihypertensive drugs (Table 12.1).

Treatment guidelines include:

- One or more antihypertensive medications may be necessary to achieve satisfactory blood pressure control.
- Adding a second drug to small or moderate doses of the first drug often results in better control with fewer side effects than using full doses of the first agent.
- Angiotensin-converting enzyme (ACE) inhibitors commonly are the first choice for therapy because they are effective and have a low incidence of side effects. They have no negative impact on carbohydrate or lipid metabolism, can slow the rate of progression of proteinuria in diabetic nephropathy, and reduce the decline in renal function.[6] Caution should be used in patients with peripheral occlusive disease because renal artery stenosis may be present, which could lead to renal decline with ACE inhibitors.
- Additional appropriate choices for initial therapy include calcium-channel blockers, indapamide, and alpha-adrenergic blockers, either alone or in combination.
- Serum potassium should be monitored during therapy with ACE inhibitors in patients with suspected hyporeninemic hypoaldosteronism (type IV renal tubular acidosis) to prevent severe hyperkalemia.
- Low doses of thiazides and beta-blockers can be used occasionally, when the preferred drugs do not control the blood pressure, with minimal

adverse effects. Although these agents are effective at lowering blood pressure, they typically worsen glucose control, exacerbate the atherogenic lipid profile, worsen peripheral vascular disease, and are associated with other adverse effects such as impotence, hypoglycemia unawareness, and hyperuricemia.

■ Dyslipidemia

Lipid abnormalities that accelerate atherosclerosis and increase the risk of cardiovascular disease are significantly more common in patients with type II diabetes than in nondiabetic individuals. In addition, central obesity associated with type II diabetes is also a risk factor for cardiovascular disease. These combined factors have resulted in cardiovascular disease becoming a major cause of morbidity and mortality in type II diabetes.

The characteristic lipid abnormalities in type II diabetes are:

- Hypertriglyceridemia due to elevated triglyceride-rich, very low-density lipoprotein (VLDL) levels and decreased high-density lipoprotein (HDL) levels
- Phenotype B pattern (excessive amounts of small, dense low-density lipoprotein [LDL] and intermediate-density lipoprotein [IDL] particles), which contribute to an increased cardiovascular risk.

Given this higher risk of premature cardiovascular disease in type II diabetes, all patients should be screened for lipid abnormalities at the initial evaluation using a fasting lipid profile to determine serum triglyceride, total cholesterol, HDL cholesterol, and LDL cholesterol levels. Shown in Table 12.2 are acceptable, borderline, and high-risk lipid levels for adults. LDL cholesterol is calculated from the formula:

TABLE 12.1 — POTENTIAL COMPLICATIONS OF ANTIHYPERTENSIVE DRUG CLASSES IN THE PATIENT WITH DIABETES

Drug	Potential Complications
Diuretics	
Potassium-losing (thiazides, loop diuretics)	Hypokalemia, hyperglycemia, dyslipidemia, impotence
Potassium-sparing	Hyperkalemia, impotence, gynecomastia
Vasodilators	Exacerbation of coronary heart disease, fluid retention
Sympathetic inhibitors	Orthostatic hypotension, impotence, depression
α-Adrenergic blockers	Orthostatic hypotension
β-Adrenergic blockers	
Nonselective	Cardiac failure, impaired insulin release with hyperglycemia, hypoglycemia unawareness, delayed recovery from hyperglycemia, impotence
Cardioselective (cardioselectivity may be lost with high doses)	Blunted symptoms of hypoglycemia, hypertension associated with hypoglycemia, hyperlipidemia, impotence
Angiotensin-converting enzyme inhibitors	Proteinuria (can occur in patients with severe bilateral renal artery stenosis), hyperkalemia, cough, leukopenia/agranulocytosis (rare)
Calcium-channel blockers	Pedal edema, constipation, heart block, negative inotropic effect (depending on agent selected)

Source: Adapted from Christlieb AR. Treating hypertension in the patient with diabetes. *Med Clin North Am.* 1982;66:1373-1388.

TABLE 12.2 — LIPID LEVELS FOR ADULTS

Risk for Adult Diabetic Patients	Cholesterol (mg/dL)	HDL Cholesterol (mg/dL)	LDL Cholesterol (mg/dL)	Triglycerides (mg/dL)
Acceptable	< 200	—	100	< 200
Borderline	200 - 239	—	100 - 129	200 - 399
High	≥ 240	≥ 35	≥ 130	≥ 400

Source: American Diabetes Association. Consensus statement: detection and management of lipid disorders in diabetes. *Diabetes Care*. 1995;18:86-93.

12

$$LDL = total\ cholesterol - HDL - (triglycerides \div 5)$$

This calculation is not accurate if the triglycerides are greater than 400 mg/dL and LDL can then be measured directly by ultracentrifugation.

Because lipid abnormalities often reflect poor glycemic control, the first treatment approach to hyperlipidemia in type II diabetes should be optimizing diabetes control with diet, exercise, and pharmacologic therapy as needed. As glycemic control improves, lipid levels also improve, particularly when insulin resistance is the underlying metabolic anomaly responsible for the lipid disorder.

Limiting calories and fat intake have proved to be highly effective in improving, but not usually normalizing, the dyslipidemia of type II diabetes. Increased intake of soluble fiber, particularly from oat and bean products, has been shown to reduce LDL cholesterol levels. The National Cholesterol Education Program (NCEP) has designed a stepped approach for restricting dietary fat and cholesterol that can be modified to incorporate specific requirements for diabetic nutrition.[7] The following guidelines should be implemented with the assistance of a registered dietitian:

- Step 1 diet guidelines: limit saturated fat intake to 8% to 10% of daily calories, with 30% of calories from total fat; limit cholesterol to < 300 mg cholesterol per day. If this approach is not adequate for meeting lipid goals, initiate Step 2.
- Step 2 diet guidelines: limit saturated fat intake to < 7% of daily calories; limit cholesterol intake to < 200 mg/day.
- If triglycerides are > 1000 mg/dL, all dietary fats should be reduced to lower circulating chylomicrons.

Recommendations for effective diet therapy for the treatment of lipid disorders in diabetes are shown in Table 12.3.

Lipid-lowering pharmacologic agents are usually necessary when the lipid profile does not normalize in response to diet, exercise, and efforts to improve glycemic control. When serum triglycerides are consistently elevated above 200 mg/dL, with or without low HDL levels, medication is warranted in addition to a low-fat diet.

- When hypertriglyceridemia is the primary lipid abnormality (triglyceride levels consistently > 200 mg/dL with or without low HDL levels): gemfibrozil (Lopid), a fibric acid derivative, is the drug of choice, 600 mg given twice daily before breakfast and dinner unless renal insufficiency coexists. This agent is particularly effective at decreasing hepatic VLDL production and enhancing the clearance of VLDL triglycerides by stimulating lipoprotein lipase (LPL). Gemfibrozil is well tolerated.

TABLE 12.3 — DIET RECOMMENDATIONS FOR THE TREATMENT OF LIPID DISORDERS IN DIABETES

- Calorie restriction for weight loss as indicated
- Total fat intake < 30% of kcal, mostly monounsaturated (eg, canola oil, olive oil)
- Saturate fat intake < 10% of total kcal
- Total cholesterol intake < 300 mg/day
- Carbohydrate intake 50% to 60% of total calories, emphasizing complex carbohydrates (at least five portions per day of fruits/vegetables); soluble fibers (legumes, oats, certain fruits/vegetables) have additional benefits on total cholesterol, LDL cholesterol level, and glycemic control
- Sodium restriction < 2400 mg/day for type II diabetic patients with hypertension

12

- When elevated LDL cholesterol is the primary lipoprotein abnormality: HMG-CoA reductase inhibitors (Mevacor, Zocor, Pravachol, Lescol) are indicated. These agents reduce cholesterol synthesis and are useful as monotherapy for the familial forms of hypercholesterolemia, or in combination with bile acid sequestrants.
- Bile acid sequestrants (Colestid, Questran) have several disadvantages in patients with diabetes. Bile binders must be taken 1 hour before or 4 hours after other oral medications so there is no interference with absorption. Bile binders also cause fairly significant constipation, and this is especially bothersome in the diabetic population because it exacerbates the constipation of diabetic gastroparesis. In addition, bile binders also can worsen hypertriglyceridemia in patients with diabetes.
- Nicotinic acid is highly effective at improving all lipoprotein parameters, although it significantly worsens glucose intolerance and is contraindicated in most patients with type II diabetes.
- Despite earlier warnings that HMG-CoA reductase inhibitors should not be used with gemfibrozil in patients with mixed disorders, they offer a safe and effective approach to diabetic patients with elevated triglycerides and LDL cholesterol values. When adding one medication to the other, creatinine phosphokinase (CPK) should be measured and liver function tests should be performed in 3 weeks and again in 6 weeks, along with a lipoprotein profile. Once a stable dose is maintained and the CPK and liver function tests are below 3 times the upper limit of normal, then monitoring these values frequently becomes unnecessary. Caution should be used if the patient is on other medications that could cause hepatitis or myositis. Lastly,

this combination should only be used in compliant patients who will not get lost to medical follow-up.

Microvascular Complications

Retinopathy, nephropathy, and neuropathy are the major microvascular complications of type II diabetes. Prevention, early detection, and aggressive treatment are essential to reduce associated morbidity and mortality. Good metabolic control has been clearly shown to prevent the development and delay the progression of these complications in type I diabetes, and comparable benefits are thought to be likely in type II diabetes.[2-3]

■ Diabetic Retinopathy

The development and progression of retinopathy depends on the duration of diabetes and the duration and severity of hyperglycemia. Because diabetic retinopathy does not cause symptoms until it has reached an advanced stage, early and frequent evaluation for vision problems is critical for patients with diabetes. The following findings also support the importance of early detection:[8-9]

- Diabetes is the leading cause of all new cases of blindness (12%).
- Loss of vision associated with diabetic retinopathy and macular edema can be reduced by at least 50% with laser photocoagulation if identified in a timely manner.

Patients must be completely informed about the possible relationship between hyperglycemia and retinopathy, stressing the importance of promptly reporting any visual symptoms. They should be aware that hypertension can worsen retinopathy and therefore be encouraged to take any antihypertensive medications that have been prescribed. Most importantly, patients should understand the potential visual complications associated with diabetic retinopathy and how to prevent or reduce the severity of these problems.

The three categories of diabetic retinopathy that are part of a continuum are:

- Nonproliferative or background
- Preproliferative
- Proliferative.

Nonproliferative

Background changes are the earliest stage of retinopathy and are characterized by microaneurysms and intraretinal "dot and blot" hemorrhages (Figure 12.1). If serous fluid leaks into the area of the maculae (where central vision originates), macular edema can occur and cause disruption in light transmission and visual acuity. Macular edema cannot be observed directly but is suggested by the presence of hard exudates close to the maculae. Any of these findings should prompt immediate referral to an ophthalmologist.

Preproliferative

Advanced background retinopathy with certain lesions is considered the preproliferative stage and indicates an increased risk of progression to proliferative retinopathy. This stage is characterized by "beading" of the retinal veins; soft exudates (also called "cotton-wool, spots that are ischemic infarcts of the inner retinal layers) (Figure 12.2); and irregular, dilated, and tortuous retinal capillaries or occasionally newly formed intraretinal vessels. Any of these signs suggests the need for further evaluation by an ophthalmologist.

Proliferative

Proliferative retinopathy is the final stage of this degenerative condition and imparts the most serious threat to vision. Neovascularization typically covers

FIGURE 12.1 — BACKGROUND DIABETIC RETINOPATHY

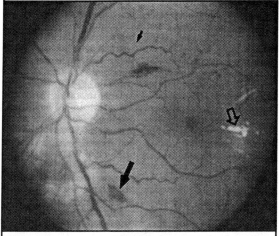

Note microaneurysm (short dark arrow), hard exudate (open arrow), and hemorrhage (long dark arrow).

Courtesy of Albert Sheffer, MD.

more than one third of the optic disk and may extend into the posterior vitreous. These fragile new vessels, which are prone to bleeding, probably develop in response to ischemia. Bleeding that occurs in the vitreous or preretinal space can cause visual symptoms such as "floaters" or "cobwebs," or retinal detachment that results from contraction of fibrous tissue. Sudden and painless vision loss usually is related to a major retinal hemorrhage.

Evaluation and Referral

Because visual acuity frequently changes in response to fluctuations in glycemic control (particularly extreme variations, eg, low-to-high and high-to-low), the reason for any vision changes should be thoroughly investigated. All patients with diabetes should

171

FIGURE 12.2 — PREPROLIFERATIVE RETINOPATHY

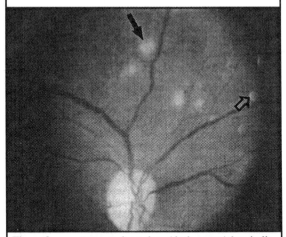

The soft or cotton wool exudate (dark arrow) has indistinct margins in contrast to the hard exudate in Figure 12.1, which has sharp margins and is brighter. The round structures with distinct margins (open arrow) are artifacts.

Courtesy of Albert Sheffer, MD.

have annual eye examinations with complete visual history, visual acuity examinations, and careful ophthalmoscopic examinations with a dilated pupil. Indications for referral to an ophthalmologist are shown in Table 12.4. Patients with type I diabetes should begin having annual eye examinations after 5 years of diabetes. Patients with type II diabetes should have annual eye examinations starting at the time of diagnosis because of the probability that glucose intolerance was present for up to 4 to 7 years before the diagnosis of diabetes.

TABLE 12.4 — REASONS TO REFER PATIENTS WITH TYPE II DIABETES MELLITUS TO AN EYE DOCTOR

High-risk Patients
Annual examinations
- Neovascularization covering more than one third of optic disk
- Vitreous or preretinal hemorrhage with any neovascularization, particularly on optic disk
- Macular edema

Symptomatic Patients
Annual examinations
- Blurry vision persisting for > 1 to 2 days when not associated with a change in blood glucose
- Sudden loss of vision in one or both eyes
- Black spots, cobwebs, or flashing lights in field of vision

Asymptomatic Patients
Annual examinations are imperative
- Hard exudates near macula
- Any preproliferative or proliferative characteristics
- Pregnancy

Source: Reprinted with permission from American Diabetes Association. *Medical Management of Non–insulin-dependent (Type II) Diabetes,* 3rd ed. Alexandria, Va: American Diabetes Association; 1994:72.

12

Treatment

Treatment of nonproliferative and preproliferative retinopathy typically involves blood glucose control and blood pressure control. The only standard treatment for background retinopathy, in addition to optimizing metabolic control and blood pressure, is photocoagulation treatment. Results of the Early Treatment Diabetic Retinopathy Study (ETDRS)[7] revealed the effectiveness of argon laser photocoagulation applied focally (eg, spot-welding the leaking microaneurysms) in treating macular edema and stabilizing vision. Photocoagulation can slow the progression of vision loss in cases of macular edema and reduce visual loss by more than 50% when used as a preventive measure to limit neovascularization and vitreous hemorrhages. Panretinal laser treatment has been proven effective[10] and is the treatment of choice for patients with proliferative retinopathy and high-risk characteristics. A scatter pattern of 1200 to 1600 burns are applied throughout the periphery of the retina, avoiding the macular area.

Vitrectomy may be required to treat retinal detachment and large vitreous hemorrhages. This procedure generally is reserved for patients with poor vision in whom the benefits outweigh the risks.

■ Diabetic Nephropathy

Over 20% of adults who have had diabetes for 20 years or more have clinically apparent nephropathy.[7] This disease is progressive, takes years to develop, and requires laboratory evaluation for early detection because it generally is asymptomatic in the early stages.

Structural and functional changes in the kidneys occur early in the course of poorly controlled diabetes but do not produce clinical symptoms. The first sign of nephropathy is microalbuminuria (30 to 300 mg albumin/24 h), which may be apparent at the time of diagnosis in patients with type II diabetes. The presence of microalbuminurea is not only a predictable marker of early diabetic nephropathy, but is also very strongly associated with coronary artery disease in patients with type II diabetes. In addition, hyperfiltration, indicated by an elevated creatinine clearance, is also a finding in early diabetic nephropathy. The important clinical point is that in this early stage of nephropathy, aggressive management may reverse or completely stabilize any abnormalities. Overt nephropathy is defined as urinary protein excretion > 0.5 g/24 h and clinical proteinuria characterized by albumin excretion rates > 300 mg (0.3 g)/24 h, typically accompanied by hypertension.[1] The following conditions play a role in the development and acceleration of renal insufficiency:

- Hypertension (virtually all patients who develop nephropathy also have hypertension [SBP > 135 mm Hg, DBP > 85 mm Hg])
- Neurogenic bladder due to hydronephrosis
- Urinary tract infection and obstruction
- Nephrotoxic drugs (nonsteroidal anti-inflammatory drugs, chronic analgesic abuse, radiocontrast dyes [should be performed only when adequate hydration and diuresis can be assured and if no other diagnostic alternatives are available]).

The final, end-stage renal disease is similar to kidney failure requiring dialysis, with two important exceptions. First, patients with diabetes often develop uremia at lower creatinine levels than patients with renal insufficiency resulting from other causes. Second, even with dialysis the prognosis for patients with diabetes is worse than that for nondiabetic patients. Patients with diabetes tend to start dialysis earlier because they develop symptoms sooner than other patients with renal disease. Therefore, a renal transplant is the preferred method of treatment, if possible, at this stage.

Evaluation

Early detection is essential. Renal function should be evaluated initally in all new patients and at yearly intervals in all adult patients with diabetes; a dipstick method is recommended for screening for microalbuminurea or determining the albumin-to-creatinine ratio.[11] Urinalysis with microscopic analysis should include urea and serum creatinine measurements; a 24-

hour or overnight specimen should be collected to test for microalbuminuria, proteinuria, and creatinine clearance. If a urinary tract infection is present it should be treated promptly before determining the significance of proteinuria. A positive result (> 30 mg protein/24 h) indicates the need for pharmacologic therapy.

Annual screening is important for patients who have negative results (particularly those without microalbuminuria and hypertension), given that certain factors can interfere transiently with this evaluation (eg, exercise, infections, fever, uncontrolled diabetes, hypertension). The mean albumin excretion of three timed urine collections can be used to establish a diagnosis of microalbuminuria if the values are equivocal.[11]

It is important for physicians to inform patients with diabetes about the relationship between high blood pressure and renal disease, and the benefits of maintaining glycemic control. Patients should be encouraged to have their blood pressure checked regularly (in addition to obtaining their own blood pressure cuff to measure blood pressure at home), take antihypertensive medications that have been prescribed, decrease their protein intake to approximately 10% of daily calories, and monitor glucose levels frequently with self-monitoring of capillary blood glucose (SMCBG) and take any other measures to improve glycemia. The importance of reporting symptoms of urinary tract infection should be emphasized, along with following proper treatment for this infection and avoiding nephrotoxic drugs.

Treatment

Treatment is aimed at early detection and prevention, focusing specifically on improving glycemic control, aggressively treating hypertension (eg, with ACE inhibitor therapy), and restricting protein intake. If proteinuria is persistent or progressive, hypertension does not respond to treatment, or serum creatinine continues to be elevated, a nephrologist should be consulted. There is also evidence that treating an elevated LDL cholesterol level may be beneficial to the diabetic kidney.

Improving Glycemic Control

Considerable evidence supports the importance of optimizing glycemic control in delaying the development and slowing the progression of diabetic nephropathy.[2-3,12] In the DCCT,[3] intensive metabolic control was associated with a decrease in the development of microalbuminuria and clinical grade proteinuria in patients with type I diabetes, with logical extrapolation to type II diabetic patients. The benefits of improved glycemia appear to be greatest before the onset of macroalbuminuria; once overt diabetic nephropathy has developed, improved glycemia has little beneficial effects on the progression of renal disease.

Current research[13] has revealed a glycemic threshold for developing microalbuminuria, establishing a glycosylated hemoglobin level of < 8% (normal is 4% to 6%) as a reasonable initial glycemic goal. The risk of developing microalbuminuria is substantially reduced at this level, with minimal risk of hypoglycemia.

Treating Hypertension

Controlling hypertension through aggressive therapeutic intervention can reduce proteinuria and considerably delay the progression of renal insufficiency. ACE inhibitors offer effective antihypertensive effects in addition to significant delaying of the progression of diabetic nephropathy to end-stage renal disease.[11] ACE inhibitors decrease proteinuria by minimizing efferent glomerular vasoconstriction and reducing glomerular hyperfiltration. In cases where the glomerular filtration rate has already declined, ACE inhibitors also can partially reverse or prevent a further

12

decrease. ACE inhibitors should be considered as first-line therapy in all normotensive and hypertensive patients with diabetes who have microalbuminuria or macroalbuminuria.

When blood pressure cannot be adequately controlled with the maximum dose of an ACE inhibitor, additional antihypertensive medications may be needed, such as calcium channel blockers, alpha-blockers (indapamide) and centrally acting agents (clonidine patch).[11] Patients with renal insufficiency and hypertension may be given a diuretic as part of the antihypertensive regimen because of related sodium and fluid retention; a loop diuretic usually is necessary if the creatinine level exceeds 2 mg/dL.

Restricting Protein Intake

Protein intake should be limited to 0.8 g/kg/day or approximately 10% of daily calories, derived primarily from lean animal and vegetable or plant sources, in patients with diabetes and evidence of nephropathy.[14] Vegetable proteins appear to have beneficial renal effects compared with animal sources and provide an important protein supplement or substitute in low-protein diets. The value of restricting protein intake in the absence of diabetic renal disease has not been clearly demonstrated. Low-protein diets can be made more palatable with a greater variety of vegetable protein sources and increased consumption of high-fiber complex carbohydrates and monounsaturated fats.[14]

■ Diabetic Neuropathy

The various diabetic neuropathies are one of the most common yet distressing long-term complications of diabetes, affecting 60% to 70% of patients with type I and type II diabetes.[8] The categories of diabetic neuropathy are shown in Table 12.5.

Symmetric Distal Neuropathy

These neuropathies develop most often in the lower extremities, causing numbness and tingling (pins-and-needles paresthesias) usually during the night. Some patients develop painful burning and stabbing symptoms that can interfere with their quality of life and may be associated with neuropathic cachexia syndrome that includes anorexia, depression, and weight loss. Treatments that have varying degrees of effectiveness, particularly for painful neuropathies, include tricyclic antidepressants, carbamazepine, phenytoin, and counterirritants such as topical capsaicin. Aspirin or propoxyphene should be prescribed as necessary for pain; narcotic analgesics generally should be avoided because of the risk of addiction with chronic use. A treatment flow chart for managing painful diabetic neuropathy is shown in Figure 12.3.

Mononeuropathy

These neuropathies can occur in virtually any cranial or peripheral nerve, are asymmetric, and have an

---

TABLE 12.5 — TYPES OF DIABETIC NEUROPATHIES

Sensorimotor Peripheral Neuropathies
- Symmetric, distal, bilateral of upper/lower extremities
- Mononeuropathies
- Diabetic amyotrophy

Autonomic Neuropathies
- Gastroparesis diabeticorum
- Diabetic diarrhea
- Neurogenic bladder
- Impaired cardiovascular reflex responses
- Impotence

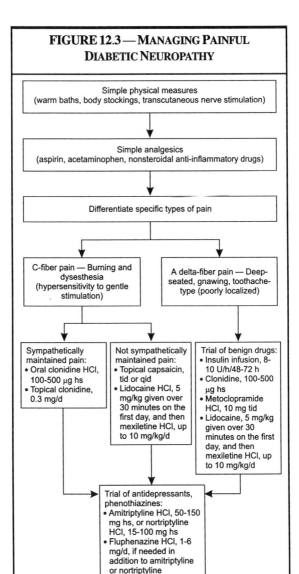

FIGURE 12.3 — MANAGING PAINFUL DIABETIC NEUROPATHY

Simple physical measures
(warm baths, body stockings, transcutaneous nerve stimulation)

↓

Simple analgesics
(aspirin, acetaminophen, nonsteroidal anti-inflammatory drugs)

↓

Differentiate specific types of pain

C-fiber pain — Burning and dysesthesia (hypersensitivity to gentle stimulation)

A delta-fiber pain — Deep-seated, gnawing, toothache-type (poorly localized)

Sympathetically maintained pain:
- Oral clonidine HCl, 100-500 μg hs
- Topical clonidine, 0.3 mg/d

Not sympathetically maintained pain:
- Topical capsaicin, tid or qid
- Lidocaine HCl, 5 mg/kg given over 30 minutes on the first day, and then mexiletine HCl, up to 10 mg/kg/d

Trial of benign drugs:
- Insulin infusion, 8-10 U/h/48-72 h
- Clonidine, 100-500 μg hs
- Metoclopramide HCl, 10 mg tid
- Lidocaine, 5 mg/kg given over 30 minutes on the first day, and then mexiletine HCl, up to 10 mg/kg/d

Trial of antidepressants, phenothiazines:
- Amitriptyline HCl, 50-150 mg hs, or nortriptyline HCl, 15-100 mg hs
- Fluphenazine HCl, 1-6 mg/d, if needed in addition to amitriptyline or nortriptyline

Modified from: Vinik AI, Holland MT, Le Beau JM, et al. Diabetic neuropathies. *Diabetes Care.* 1992;15:1926.

abrupt onset. Cranial mononeuropathies are the most common, particularly the third and sixth, causing extraocular muscle motor paralysis and peripheral palsies. Patients can develop palsies involving the peroneal (foot drop), median, and ulner nerves. Spontaneous recovery over 3 to 6 months is typical. Patients with diabetes are more prone to developing compression neuropathies such as carpal tunnel syndrome.

Diabetic Amyotrophy

This neuropathy often is asymmetric, is more common in men, and is characterized by severe pain, muscle wasting in the pelvic girdle and quadricep muscles, and mild sensory involvement. This condition usually is self-limiting, with complete recovery typically occurring in 6 to 12 months. Treatment is focused on maintaining glycemic control and symptomatic relief using physical therapy and analgesics.

Gastroparesis

This neuropathy should be suspected in patients with nausea, vomiting, early satiety, abdominal distention, and bloating following a meal, and is secondary to delayed emptying and retention of gastric contents. The delay in gastric emptying usually is asymptomatic, although glycemic control can be affected. Postprandial hypoglycemia and delayed hyperglycemia develop when the balance between exogenous insulin administration and nutrient absorption is disrupted because of gastric stasis. Therefore, gastroparesis should be considered even in the absence of gastrointestinal symptoms in a patient who suddenly develops unexplainable poor glycemic control after having had satisfactory control.

Primary treatment is focused on optimizing glucose control with insulin; secondary treatment involves dietary modifications in the form of a low-fat, low-residue diet.[15] When patients remain symptomatic despite

12

these measures, treatment with the following prokinetic agents is recommended:[15]

- Erythromycin lactobionate 1.5 to 3.0 mg/kg body weight IV every 6 to 8 hours (acute treatment, effective in eliminating residue from stomach); common side effects are nausea and vomiting.
- Oral treatment with cisapride, 10 to 20 mg before meals and at bedtime (enhances gastric emptying through serotoninergic mechanisms, effective in acute conditions); minimal side effects (abdominal cramping, frequent bowel movements); long-term use may cause hyperprolactinemia, galactorrhea, menstrual irregularities.
- Oral metoclopramide HCl is discouraged because of adverse reactions (nervousness, anxiety, dystonic effects, and the potential for irreversible tardive dyskinesia).
- Oral treatment with domperidone, a peripheral dopamine antagonist (FDA approval pending), 10 to 20 mg 3 to 4 times daily (accelerates gastric emptying); minimal side effects (abdominal cramping, frequent bowel movements) and rare adverse reactions (hyperprolactinemia, galactorrhea).

■ Diabetic Diarrhea

Intermittent diarrhea may alternate with constipation and can be difficult to treat. Diabetic diarrhea is a diagnosis of exclusion. High fiber intake can be helpful, along with diphenoxylate (Lomotil), loperamide (Immodium), or clonidine. Small intestine stasis contributes to bacterial overgrowth, causing diarrhea. Treatment with one of the following antibiotics for 10 to 14 days is recommended:[15]

- Doxycycline hyclate, 100 mg every 12 hours
- Amoxicillin trihydrate, 250 mg every 6 hours
- Metronidazole, 250 mg every 6 hours
- Ciprofloxacin HCl, 250 mg every 12 hours.

A trial of pancreatic enzymes is also recommended to rule out exocrine pancreatic insufficiency. In many instances, tincture of opium is the only medication that can help the patient live a nearly normal daily life.

■ Neurogenic Bladder

Frequent small voidings and incontinence that may progress to urinary retention characterize this neuropathy. Confirmation of this diagnosis requires demonstration of cystometric abnormalities and large residual urine volume. Most medical treatment is inadequate, although scheduling frequent voidings every 3 to 4 hours combined with bethanechol 10 to 50 mg 3 to 4 times daily supplemented by small doses of phenoxybenzamine may be helpful. Surgical intervention may be necessary if patients do not respond to pharmacologic therapy because chronic urinary retention can lead to urinary tract infection.

■ Impaired Cardiovascular Reflexes

Orthostatic hypotension and fixed tachycardia are the most disturbing and disabling autonomic symptoms. Typical treatment of orthostatic hypotension includes elevating the head of the bed, compression stockings for lower limbs and torso, supplementary salt intake, and the use of fludrocortisone (0.05 mg initially with gradual increases of 0.1 mg up to 0.5 to 1 mg). This pharmacologic therapy should be used cautiously in patients with cardiac disease because it causes sodium and water retention and may precipitate congestive heart failure.

■ Impotence in Men

Erectile dysfunction, or impotence, is defined as the consistent inability for a man to get or keep an erection for satisfactory sexual intercourse. It is a couples' disorder, as both patient and partner suffer. Diabetic impotence is usually caused by circulatory and nervous system abnormalities and is a very common complaint in the male diabetic population. The classic clinical picture includes a patient with normal sexual desire but the inability to physically act on that desire. If a patient tells you he has morning erections, he can masturbate without problems, or his libido is abnormally low, look for other causes of impotence such as psychological problems or a low androgen state. Orgasm and ejaculation are usually normal. Even if the patient does not have any psychological problems that could cause the impotence, he may develop a secondary psychological fear of failure that could complicate the clinical picture.

The diagnosis can be made in most cases by a good sexual, psychosocial, and medical history, a physical examination, and laboratory tests. A testosterone level should be drawn to rule out a low androgen state, which is rarely a cause for impotence.

Hyperprolactinemia is also an uncommon cause of impotence. Hemochromatosis is a condition that is underdiagnosed and is associated with impotence and glucose intolerance. Serum iron stores, including ferritin levels, are abnormally high in this disorder. If the patient has femoral bruits and/or peripheral occlusive disease, then a vascular workup may help identify the cause of impotence.

Make sure the patient is not on any medications that can cause impotence such as beta-blockers and thiazide diuretics. ACE inhibitors, calcium-channel blockers, and alpha-blockers do not generally cause impotence.

Despite the prevalence of this disorder, nearly all patients can be successfully treated with either nonsurgical or surgical means. Yohimbine HCl, an alpha$_2$-adrenergic blocking agent, has been widely used as a nonhormonal medication for the treatment of impotence. However, there has been a consistent lack of data to show that it is more effective than placebo.

Testosterone given by injection or via a scrotal or skin patch is only indicated when the serum testosterone levels are low on several occasions. If there might be binding protein abnormalities, then a free testosterone level is indicated. As mentioned above, a low testosterone state is rarely a cause of impotence.

Vacuum constrictor devices are a new and viable therapeutic option for diabetic patients with impotence. No surgery or injections are required, patient acceptance is excellent, and there are few side effects. The majority of these external penile devices have a vacuum chamber that goes over the penis, a vacuum pump that creates negative pressure within the chamber allowing for engorgement of the penis with blood, and a constrictor band that is placed over the base of the penis when tumescence is achieved. Side effects are minor and include ecchymoses, hematomas, and pain. These devices are effective in men with both total and partial impotence. Many patients discover that they do not need the device after a brief period of time, which indicates that a fear of failure or other psychological problems were the initial cause of impotence.

Intracavernosal injection of vasoactive agents such as papaverine or prostaglandins can be self administered and work by relaxing corporal smooth muscle. Intracavernosal injections will work best in patients with diabetic impotence whose arterial inflow and corporal veno-occlusion mechanism is normal. Side effects include the formation of painless fibrotic nodules within the corpora cavernosa and priapism. Titration guidelines should be followed when initiating therapy. Despite the route of administration, patient acceptance is also good.

Penile prostheses represent an excellent surgical option for the treatment of impotence. The options range from simple malleable or semirigid prostheses to inflatable devices that use hydraulic principles to inflate and deflate the penis when desired. Surgical complications are very low, especially when the patient's glycemic control has been acceptable prior to surgery. With the availability of intracavernosal injections and vacuum devices, surgery has become a third-line treatment of choice.

Diabetic Foot Disorders

More than half of all nontraumatic amputations in the United States occur in individuals with diabetes, and the majority of these could have been prevented with proper foot care. Efforts aimed at prevention, early detection, and treatment of diabetic foot disorders can have a significant impact on the incidence of these problems.

■ Detection and Treatment

The physician and patient must diligently examine the feet on a regular basis for signs of redness or trauma. Lack of pain, position, and vibratory sensations caused by neuropathy, associated deformities, and vascular ischemia can faciliate the development of foot lesions. Foot pressure that is abnormally distributed predisposes a neuropathic patient to pressure ischemia and skin breakdown. Autonomic neuropathy causes decreased sweating and dry skin that can result in cracked, thickened skin that is susceptible to infection and ulceration.

Pressure perception can be assessed using the Semmes Weinstein monofilaments, which are available in three thicknesses: 1-g fiber (SW 4.17 rating), 10-g fiber (SW 5.07 rating), and 75-g fiber (SW 6.10 rating). The following evaluation procedure has been recommended:[16]

Place the monofilament against the skin and apply pressure to different areas of the bottom of the foot until the filament buckles. The patient should be able to feel the monofilament when it buckles and identify the location being tested. The 5.07 thickness monofilament, which is equivalent to 10-g of linear pressure, detects the presence or absence of protective sensation and is useful for identifying a foot at risk for ulceration and in need of special care.

Daily inspection of feet can help detect early skin lesions, and proper footwear can minimize the development of foot problems. Patients should be taught to cut toenails straight across and not trim calluses themselves, regularly wash their feet with warm water and mild soap, and avoid going barefoot or wearing constricting shoes. Minor wounds that are not infected can be treated with mild antiseptic solution, daily dressing changes, and foot rest. Patient guidelines for care of the diabetic foot are shown in Table 12.6.

Podiatrists should be consulted for assistance with more serious foot problems and for regular nail and callus care in high-risk individuals. If an ulcer develops, the skin must be debrided and the pressure alleviated; infections should be treated promptly with medications appropriate for the offending organism. Healing is facilitated by bed rest with foot elevation and the use of an orthopedic walking cast to relieve pressure but allow mobility. Intravenous antibiotics, surgical debridement, distal arterial revascularization, and local foot-sparing surgery may help prevent amputation in cases of seriously infected foot ulcers.

REFERENCES

1. Davidson MB. *Diabetes Mellitus: Diagnosis and Treatment*, 3rd ed. New York: Churchill Livingstone; 1991.

2. Reichard P, Nilsson BY, Rosenqvist U. The effect of long-term intensified insulin treatment on the develop-

TABLE 12.6 — CARE OF THE DIABETIC FOOT

- Wash feet daily and dry carefully, especially between the toes. (Same after shower, jacuzzi, or swimming.)

- Inspect your feet daily for blisters, cuts, scratches, and areas of possible infection. Look between the toes! A mirror can help you see the bottom of your feet and between toes. If it is not possible for you to inspect your feet, seek the help of a family member or friend.

- If your feet feel cold at night, wear socks. Do not apply hot water bottles or heating pads.

- Avoid extreme temperatures for your feet. Test bath water with your hand to ensure that it is not too hot, and be extremely careful of hot pavement or concrete in the summer.

- Inspect your shoes daily for foreign objects, nail points, torn linings, or other problems.

- Change socks daily, wear properly fitting socks, and avoid holes or mended socks. "THOR-LO" socks have extra padding in heel and ball of foot for better shock absorption (available in sporting goods stores).

- All shoes should be comfortable at the time of purchase. Do not depend on shoes to break in. Wear them only 1 hour the first day, and only in the house. Check your feet for blisters, and then slowly increase the wearing time.

- Do not wear sandals with thongs between the toes, and never wear shoes without socks.

- Never walk barefoot, not even in the house, because of danger from stepping on pins, needles, tacks, glass, or other items on the floor.

- Do not use chemical agents to remove corns or calluses, and do not cut them yourself. Consult your podiatrist and be sure to let him/her know you are diabetic.

- Toenails should be cut straight across. If you have trouble or questions about them, see your podiatrist.

- Infections from cuts, scratches, blisters, etc, can cause significant problems in diabetics, and a podiatrist or physician should be seen when infection occurs. If you experience flu-like symptoms, or increased blood sugars, be sure to check your feet.

13. Do not smoke!

Reference: Goldman F, Gibbons G, Kruse-Edelmann I. Limb salvage techniques. In: *The High Risk Foot in Diabetes Mellitus*. New York: Churchill Livingstone; 1990.

ment of microvascular complications of diabetes mellitus. *N Engl J Med.* 1993;329:304-309.

3. The Diabetes Control and Complications Trial Research Group. The effect of intensive treatment of diabetes on the development and progression of long-term complications in insulin-dependent diabetes mellitus. *N Engl J Med.* 1993;329:977-986.

4. American Diabetes Association. Consensus statement: detection and management of lipid disorders in diabetes. *Diabetes Care.* 1995;18:86-93.

5. Edelman SV, White D, Henry RR. Intensive insulin therapy for patients with type II diabetes. *Curr Opin Endocrinol Diab.* 1995;2:333-340.

6. Lewis E, Hunsicker LG, Bain RP, Rohde RD. The effect of angiotensin-converting enzyme inhibition on diabetic nephropathy. *N Engl J Med.* 1993;329:1456-1462.

7. Early Treatment Diabetic Retinopathy Study Research Group. Photocoagulation for diabetic macular edema: ETDRS report no. 1. *Ophthalmology.* 1985;103;1796-1806.

8. American Diabetes Association. *Medical Management of Non–insulin-dependent (Type II) Diabetes,* 3rd ed. Alexandria, Va: American Dibaetes Association; 1994.

9. American Diabetes Association. *Diabetes 1996 Vital Statistics.* Alexandria, Va: American Diabetes Association; 1996.

10. Diabetic Retinopathy Study Research Group. Indications for photocoagulation treatment of diabetic retinopathy, DRS report no. 14. *Int Ophthalmol Clin.* 1987;27:239-253.

11. Karlsson FO, Garber AJ. Prevention and treatment of diabetic nephropathy: role of angiotensin-converting enzyme inhibitors. *Endocr Pract.* 1996;2:215-219.

12. UK Prospective Diabetes Study. VIII. Study design, progress, and performance. *Diabetologia.* 1991;34:877-890.

13. Krowlewski AS, Laffel LM, Krolewski M, Quinn M, Warram JH. Glycosylated hemoglobin and the risk of microalbuminuria in patients with insulin-dependent diabetes mellitus. *N Engl J Med.* 1995;332:1251-1255.

14. Mudaliar SR, Henry RR. Role of glycemic control and protein restriction in clinical management of diabetic kidney disease. *Endocr Pract.* 1996;2:220-226.

15. Prather CM. Evaluating and managing GI dysfunction in diabetes. *Contemp Intern Med.* 1996;8:47-54.

16. Peragallo-Dittko V, ed. *A Core Curriculum for Diabetes Education,* 2nd ed. Chicago: American Association of Diabetes Educators; 1993.

17. Goldman F, Gibbons G, Kruse-Edelmann I. Limb salvage techniques. In: *The High Risk Foot in Diabetes Mellitus.* New York: Churchill Livingstone; 1990.

13 Resources

DIRECTORY OF DIABETES
ORGANIZATIONS

**American Association of Diabetes
Educators (AADE)**
444 N. Michigan Avenue, Suite 1240
Chicago, IL 60611
312/644-2233 or 800/338-3633
800-TEAMUP4 (Diabetes Educator Access Line)

AADE is a multidisciplinary organization, with state
and regional chapters, for health professionals involved in diabetes patient education. The organization sponsors a certification program for diabetes
educators and provides grants, scholarships, and
awards for educational research and teaching activities. AADE's annual meeting features continuing
education programs on diabetes treatment and education. The organization also features a Diabetes
Educator Access Line to help people with diabetes
locate diabetes education services in their area.

Publications: AADE publishes a bimonthly journal,
The Diabetes Educator; curriculum guides; consensus statements; self-study programs; and other print
and nonprint resources for diabetes educators.

American Diabetes Association (ADA)
ADA National Service Center
1660 Duke Street
Alexandria, VA 22314
703/549-1500 or 800/232-3472

ADA is both a professional association and a private, nonprofit, voluntary organization with state and local affiliates and chapters. It serves people with diabetes and their families and friends, as well as health professionals and research scientists involved in diabetes-related activities. The organization funds diabetes research and education activities; sponsors educational programs, including an annual meeting, postgraduate courses, consensus meetings, and special symposia; administers a recognition program for diabetes outpatient education; develops professional guidelines for diabetes care; and advocates for diabetes issues in the legislative and public health arenas. Local ADA affiliates often sponsor educational programs and support groups for persons with diabetes and their families.

Publications: ADA publishes monthly and quarterly magazines for patients, including *Diabetes Forecast*; professional journals focusing on basic and clinical research, including *Diabetes*, *Diabetes Care*, *Diabetes Spectrum*, and *Diabetes Reviews*; other publications, including cookbooks, meal planing guides, pamphlets, brochures, and books for patients; and clinical manuals, nutritional guides, audiovisuals, statistical reports, and curriculum guides for professionals.

DIABETES RESEARCH AND TRAINING CENTERS (DRTCS)

The National Institute of Diabetes and Digestive and Kidney Diseases supports six DRTCs:
Einstein/Montefiore DRTC
1575 Blondell Avenue, Suite 200
Bronx, NY 10461
718/405-8271

Indiana University DRTC
Regenstrief Institute, 5th Floor
250 University Boulevard, Room 122
Indianapolis, IN 46202
317/278-0908

Michigan DRTC
University of Michigan Medical Centers
1331 E. Ann Street
Ann Arbor, MI 48109-0201
313/763-5730

University of Chicago DRTC
Center for Research in Medical Education
and Health Care
5841 S. Maryland Avenue, MC 6091
Chicago, IL 60637
773/753-1310

Vanderbilt University DRTC
Vanderbilt Medical Center
315 Medical Arts Building
1211 21st Avenue South
Nashville, TN 37212-2230
615/936-1149

Washington University DRTC
Diabetes Education Center
660 S. Euclid, Campus Box 8212
St. Louis, MO 63110
314/362-8290

13

These centers offer continuing education, seminars, and workshops on diabetes management for health-care professionals; an array of tested evaluation and assessment instruments; professional expertise in developing and implementing diabetes programs in a variety of settings; and patient referral. DRTCs are located at major medical centers affiliated with universities.

Publications: Individual centers produce a variety of educational materials, including audiovisuals for health-care professionals. For additional information about DRTC materials and programs, contact individual centers listed above.

Division of Diabetes Translation, Centers for Disease Control and Prevention (CDC)
National Center for Chronic Disease
Prevention and Health Promotion
TISB Mail Stop K-13
4770 Buford Highway NE
Atlanta, GA 30341-3724
770/488-5080

An agency of the Public Health Service, Department of Health and Human Services, CDC develops public health approaches to reduce the burden of diabetes in the United States. The agency supports diabetes control programs in 26 states and one territory; carries out state and national surveillance activities to assess diabetes prevalence, impact, and possible contributing factors; develops consensus guidelines for clinical and public health practice; supports community-based preventive programs for minority populations and the elderly; and coordinates Federal activities concerned with translating research findings into clinical practice, including issues related to cost and reimbursement practices, disability, and quality of life.

Publications: CDC distributes a practice manual for primary-care practitioners and a companion guide for patients, surveillance reports, and guidelines on patient education, educational reimbursement, and maternal and child health. State programs have produced patient and professional publications.

US Indian Health Services (IHS)
IHS Headquarters West
Central Diabetes Program
5300 Homestead Road NE
Albuquerque, NM 87110
505/248-4182

An agency of the Public Health Service, Department of Health and Human Services, IHS supports 17 model Diabetes Health Care Programs serving Native Americans and Alaskans. These programs develop and evaluate effective and culturally accepted prevention and treatment methods for diabetes and its complications. Diabetes control officers in each IHS region provide surveillance, training, and other services to promote the use of techniques recommended by the program.

Publications: The model programs and the IHS produce culturally relevant publications for native populations, including nutrition guides, complication-specific educational materials, and guides for professionals. Publications are available only to persons working with Native Americans or Alaskan populations.

13

International Diabetes Center (IDC)
3800 Park Nicollet Boulevard
Minneapolis, MN 55416
612/993-3393

A division of the Park Nicollet Medical Foundation, IDC offers education classes for people with diabetes and training programs for health professionals.

The programs for health professionals focus on team management of diabetes. IDC also provides inpatient and outpatient treatment services in adult and pediatric clinics, supports clinical research to assess new diabetes care systems and approaches, conducts psychosocial research, and supports a network of IDC satellite centers that offer specialized programs in diabetes. The IDC has been designated as a World Health Organization Collaborating Center for Diabetes Education and Training.

Publications: The organization publishes *Living Well with Diabetes*, a quarterly magazine for people with diabetes. Other publications include management and nutrition guides for patients, low-literacy patient education booklets, guides for health professionals, audiovisuals, and general publications related to chronic health problems and nutrition. For publications/mail order pharmacy services: Chronimed; PO Box 47945; Minneapolis, MN 55447-9727; 800/876-6540 or 612/546-1146.

International Diabetes Federation (IDF)
1 Rue DeFacqz
1000 Brussels, Belgium
322/538-5511

IDF collaborates with more than 100 member associations in over 80 countries, the World Health Organization, and other affiliated organizations and individuals to ensure that people with diabetes receive quality treatment and education services.

Publications: IDF publishes a newsletter, a journal entitled *IDF Bulletin, The Directory 1991: A Guide to the Activities of Member Diabetes Associations*, as well as other publications.

International Diabetic Athletes Association (IDAA)
1647 West Bethany Home Road #B
Phoenix, AZ 85015
602/433-2113 or 800/898-IDAA (800/898-4322)
Fax: 602/433-9331
e-mail: idaa@getnet.com

IDAA is a nonprofit, membership organization for persons with diabetes who participate in fitness activities at all levels. The organization sponsors workshops, conferences, and other events. It offers educational programs for active individuals with diabetes, their families, and friends. IDAA also offers educational programs to diabetes educators, coaches, school nurses, recreation workers, and other professionals who interact with people with diabetes in a recreational setting. The organization's board of directors includes well-known athletes with diabetes, physicians, and other health professionals who are experts in diabetes and sports.

Publications: IDAA publishes the quarterly newsletter, *The Challenge*, which includes helpful articles about managing diabetes during athletic activities and stories about people with diabetes who participate in sports events.

Joslin Diabetes Center
One Joslin Place
Boston, MA 02215
617/732-2400

13

The Joslin Diabetes Center offers inpatient and outpatient treatment, education, and other support services to adults and children with diabetes; provides professional medical education; sponsors camps for children with diabetes; and supports research to improve treatment and find a cure for diabetes and its complications. The center is affiliated with Harvard Medical School and a number of hospitals in the Boston area and operates affiliated clinics in several states. The Joslin Diabetes Center is one of six Diabetes Endocrinology Research Centers supported by the National Institute of Diabetes and Digestive Kidney Diseases.

Publications: Joslin produces a variety of educational materials for patients and professionals, including manuals, nutrition guides, materials for children with diabetes, and films. *The Joslin Magazine* is issued quarterly to members of the Joslin Society.

Juvenile Diabetes Foundation (JDF) International
120 Wall Street, 19th Floor
New York, NY 10005
212/889-7575
800/223-1138

JDF is a private, nonprofit, voluntary organization with chapters throughout the world. JDF raises funds to support research on the cause, cure, treatment, and prevention of diabetes and its complications. The organization awards research grants for laboratory and clinical investigations and sponsors a variety of career development and research training programs for new and established investigators. JDF also sponsors international workshops and conferences for biomedical researchers. Individual chapters offer support groups and other activities for families.

Publications: JDF publishes the quarterly journal *Countdown* and a series of patient education brochures about insulin-dependent and non–insulin-dependent diabetes.

**National Diabetes Information
Clearinghouse (NDIC)**
1 Information Way
Bethesda, MD 20892-3560
301/654-3327

NDIC is a service of the National Institute of Diabetes and Digestive and Kidney Diseases, which is the government's lead agency for diabetes research. The clearinghouse functions as an information, educational, and referral resource for health professionals, people with diabetes, and the general public.

Publications: NDIC offers a variety of publications for use by the general public, people with diabetes, and health professionals. Publications include guides for patients and professionals, bibliographies, reports, and fact sheets. The clearinghouse also publishes the newsletter *Diabetes Dateline* and maintains the diabetes subfile of the Combined Health Information Database, available through BRS Online.

National Eye Institute (NEI)
National Eye Health Education Program
Building 31, Room 6A32
31 Center Drive, MSC-2510
Bethesda, MD 20892-2510
800/869-2020
301/496-5248

13

NEI, one of the National Institutes of Health, supports basic and clinical research to develop effective treatments for diabetic eye disease. The institute's National Eye Health Education Program promotes public and professional awareness of the importance of early diagnosis and treatment of diabetic eye disease.

Publications: NEI produces patient and professional education materials related to diabetic eye disease and its treatment, including literature for patients, guides for health professionals, and education kits for community health workers and for pharmacists.

Pennsylvania Diabetes Academy
777 East Park Drive, or PO Box 8820
Harrisburg, PA 17105-8820
717/558-7750, ext. 271
800/228-7823 (in PA only) (AA Medical Society)

The academy is a nonprofit organization affiliated with the Pennsylvania Medical Society. It operates as a cooperative venture with the state's Department of Health and the Pennsylvania Diabetes Task Force offering education, training, and consultation services to health-care professionals in the state of Pennsylvania.

Publications: Materials available from the academy include a newsletter, self-study modules for physicians, and low-literacy teaching aids for diabetes educators.

Taking Control of Your Diabetes
149 7th Street
Del Mar, CA 92014
619/755-5683 (office)
619/755-6854 (fax)
website: www.tcoyd.com

Taking Control of Your Diabetes is a nonprofit organization dedicated to promoting advocacy programs for people with diabetes. The two main goals of the organization are to (1) educate people with diabetes about how to live longer by learning about their condition, and (2) educate patients to be self-advocates and work within their health-care program to get the help they need to maintain a high standard of care.

13

INDEX

Note: Page numbers in *italics* indicate figures;
page numbers followed by t indicate tables.

206

212

214